VET CLINIC
CATS

DEDICATION

*I unreservedly
dedicate this book to my wife, Jane,
and our son, Thomas, for their
ceaseless help and support in all
that I do.*

Commissioning Editor: Julian Brown
Project Editor: Tarda Davison-Aitkins
Creative Director: Keith Martin
Executive Art Director: Mark Winwood
Picture Research: Zoë Holtermann
Designer: Les Needham
Production Controller: Lee Sargent

First published in Great Britain in 2000
by Hamlyn, a division of
Octopus Publishing Group Limited
2–4 Heron Quays, London E14 4JP

First published in paperback in 2002

Copyright © 2000, 2002 Octopus Publishing Group Limited

ISBN 0 600 60729 1

A catalogue record for this book is available from
the British Library

Printed in Hong Kong

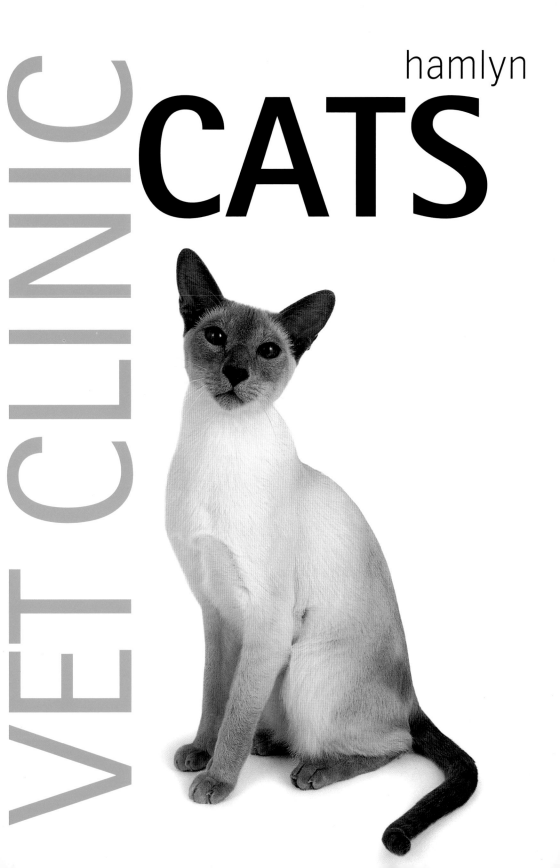

VET CLINIC

hamlyn
CATS

vet clinic

CATS

contents

Introduction

The purpose of this book is to help you to care for your cat. It describes the symptoms, causes and treatments of many of the more common medical problems that a cat owner is likely to see. To make it easier to look up specific problems, the book is divided into sections such as 'The skin', 'Movement' and 'Breathing and circulation'. Tips are given on any action you as an owner can take to help your cat, and an urgency indicator for each condition or disease tells you how important it is to seek treatment from a vet. There is also a chapter on 'Accidents and emergencies' to help you if you ever find yourself in a position where you need to give first aid to a cat.

Many medical problems are caused by the attitude of owners to their cats, and can be avoided by ensuring that a cat has a good diet, good exercise and by the owner being aware of early symptoms of illnesses. Common sense is essential in all animal husbandry, and you should take your cat to the vet for a check-up on a regular basis. Your vet will welcome any questions concerning the health and wellbeing of your cat, and will be happy to explain medical conditions – their causes, treatment and prevention – to you. Vets understand the importance of educating the cat owner, as this leads to healthier and better treated cats.

You should ensure that your cat is regularly wormed and vaccinated against the commonly occurring diseases in your area. Neutering, too, is worth considering if you do not intend to breed from your cat, as many diseases are only seen in 'entire' cats. Entire toms and queens can cause problems to both owners and their neighbours with antisocial behaviour. The unwanted kittens of these cats often end up with rescue organisations who struggle to find good, long-term homes for them. It is highly irresponsible to allow cats that have not been neutered to wander.

One of the most important ways to keep your cat healthy is to feed her a balanced, good quality diet. The main components of a balanced diet are proteins, vitamins, minerals, carbohydrates, fats and fibre. A cat fed on a properly balanced diet will be in good condition and will be able to fight off infections and disease more easily and so lead a long, active and healthy life. A whole range of complete diets for all life stages and lifestyles of cats is now easily available.

It is very important that your cat is not overweight, as obesity is linked to many problems and disorders, and an obese cat is far more likely to suffer from certain diseases. Your vet can advise you if you are concerned about your cat's weight.

Most of the treatments given in this book relate to 'normal' veterinary techniques. These are techniques taught to all vets during their training, and have served vets, and the pets for which they care, well over the years. Today, some vets are exploring other techniques and methods of treating animals. Some are now turning to what is termed a holistic approach, where the whole animal is considered, rather than simply the condition(s) that the animal is exhibiting.

One approach that vets are increasingly taking to improve the health of animals is homeopathy. This is a very complicated science, in which the vet administers extremely tiny amounts of substances that are known, in excess, to cause the problem from which the cat is suffering. The mechanism by which homeopathy works is not very well understood, but more and more people are turning to it as an alternative form of treatment. The fact that it does work, often with astonishing effect, ensures that more interest will be taken in this area of veterinary medicine in the future. Where relevant, this book lists some homeopathic treatments that may help a cat suffering from a particular disorder. If you are interested in having your pet treated homeopathically, talk it over with your vet, or if your vet appears to be cynical about the subject, contact another vet who has a genuine interest in homeopathy.

This book is not a substitute for taking a sick cat for to the vet. If your cat shows any signs of illness, it is highly recommended that you see a vet as soon as possible, as delay in some cases can mean the difference between your cat making a speedy and full recovery, or suffering a long and painful disease and, in some cases, death.

Remember: if your cat is unwell, always seek the advice of a vet as soon as possible.

Please note that throughout this book I have referred to the cat as 'she' but the text applies equally to both male and female cats (except where stated and in the chapters on problems in queens and male cat problems).

I would like to express my thanks and gratitude to Chris Charlesworth, MRCVS, and all of his staff - vets, nurses, and support workers - and his clients and patients for their help in the production of this book.

James McKay

Breathing and circulation

The respiratory system

The respiratory system supplies oxygen to the cat's body. Oxygen forms the basis of all chemical reactions inside the body, so without oxygen, or with insufficient oxygen, the cat's body would be unable to function. The cat's respiratory system has another, equally vital, role – thermo-regulation, or the control of body temperature. Any problems with the cat's respiratory system can therefore have serious effects on the cat's health.

Air breathed in through the mouth and nose passes down the trachea or windpipe into the lungs, where oxygen is taken in and carbon dioxide is passed out of the body. The trachea consists of a cylindrical tube lined with rings of tough material, called cartilage, and these rings help prevent the trachea from collapsing during normal breathing. The trachea passes into the thorax or chest cavity and then branches into smaller tubes, known as bronchi, which themselves branch, within the cat's lungs, into smaller tubes known as bronchioles. At the end of the bronchioles is a large number of alveoli, where carbon dioxide is passed out of the body's system, while oxygen is taken in. The thorax and the lungs are lined with pleura, which are thin membranes. When these membranes become inflamed, the cat's breathing becomes painful and difficult; this condition is known as pleurisy.

Small particles of debris, as well as airborne bacteria, often enter the respiratory system, but the cells lining the trachea and bronchi produce mucus, and this sticky substance helps to trap debris and airborne contaminants, stopping them from getting too far into the respiratory system. The airways also have tiny, finger-like projections, known as cilia, which physically move contaminants away. The build-up of these contaminants, along with the mucus that has trapped them, results in coughing, which expels the mucus and debris from the cat's body.

The respiratory system works together with the body's blood supply (circulatory system, see p.14). Blood from the heart is pumped to the lungs in an artery called the pulmonary artery. The lungs pass oxygen into the blood and the oxygenated blood is carried back into the heart. From there, the heart pumps the oxygenated blood around the body.

Chronic bronchial disease (Bronchitis)

Inflammation of the lining of the airways, leading to excess mucus being produced, which reduces the space available in the airways for the passage of air. Cats kept by owners who smoke are more likely to suffer from bronchitis than those whose owners do not. If this problem recurs, it can lead to permanent damage to the cat's respiratory system, in the same way as cigarette smoke and other pollution can damage the respiratory system of humans.

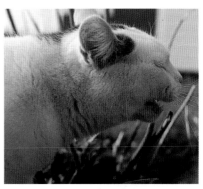

A cat which is experiencing coughing bouts may well be suffering from a bronchial infection.

URGENCY INDICATOR

Never ignore any symptoms of a possible bronchial infection, even if mild. Seek veterinary advice.

Symptoms

Persistent coughing, especially where mucus is coughed up by the cat; rapid exhaustion, following or during normal exercise, and an increase in the breathing rate (a cat's normal breathing or respiratory rate is between 10 and 30 breaths per minute).

DIAGNOSING BRONCHITIS

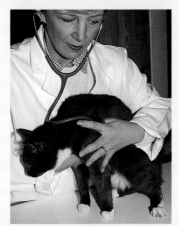

Physical examination will normally diagnose the problem, followed by X-ray examinations and laboratory analysis of mucus.

COST

In many cases of chronic bronchial disease, long-term therapy may be necessary, and this could prove expensive. Often it will be necessary for the vet to try out various combinations of drugs on the cat to find the best combination.

Underlying causes

The usual cause is long-term exposure to polluted air. As the condition is of a long-term nature, older cats (from middle age onwards) are more prone to chronic bronchial disease. Obesity also tends to make cats more prone to this disease (and many others).

Owner action

You can help to relieve the cat's breathing problems by taking her into a steamy atmosphere, such as a bathroom where a large, hot bath has recently been run. The steam will reduce congestion. If your cat suffers from bronchitis, avoid letting her out in very cold conditions, as the cold air is likely to irritate her airways.

Treatment

Any cat severely affected by chronic bronchial disease is likely to require long-term therapy. Treatment will normally consist of antibiotics to control any infection, along with drugs to reduce the production and build-up of mucus.

Rhinitis

Inflammation of the cat's nasal passages, a common symptom of cat flu (see p.11).

Symptoms
A discharge from the nose, together with bouts of sneezing.

Underlying causes
Bacterial or fungal infection can cause this condition. Where the discharge is from one nostril only (known as a unilateral discharge), this usually indicates a fungal infection or trauma. Where the discharge is from both nostrils (a bilateral discharge), this usually indicates a viral or bacterial infection. The fungus is usually *Aspergillus fumigatus*, also responsible for the disease aspergillosis in birds as well as man. In an *Aspergillus fumigatus* infection, the nasal discharge will be thick and green, and may persist for a long time – often months. Rhinitis can also be caused by foreign bodies in the nasal cavity or a nasal tumour, and it can be one of the symptoms of cat flu (see p.11).

Owner action
Keep the cat calm, and do not allow her to exert herself, and always obtain veterinary treatment as soon as possible.

Treatment
If the underlying cause is bacterial infection, the vet will prescribe a course of antibiotics. The whole course should be completed as directed. A fungal infection will be treated with anti-fungal drugs. If the problem is caused by a blockage, surgery may be required to remove it. If a cancer is the cause, the vet will advise you on the best treatment.

DIAGNOSING RHINITIS

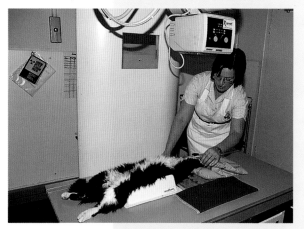

Laboratory analysis of the nasal discharge to diagnose the underlying problem. If a blockage is suspected, the vet will do a physical examination and if the problem still cannot be seen, X-ray examinations may be necessary.

RELATED CONDITIONS WHICH MAY PRODUCE SIMILAR SYMPTOMS

Sinusitis, the inflammation of the mucous membranes in the nasal cavity. This can be treated with antibiotics. *i*

◔ COST
Depends upon the underlying cause. Surgery will be more expensive than antibiotics or anti-fungal drugs.

Feline respiratory disease

HOMEOPATHIC TREATMENT:

Peruvian bark and phosphate of iron will help the cat to recover from the debilitating effects of cat flu. Phosphate of iron will relieve the symptoms of sinusitis (the inflammation of the mucous membranes in the nasal cavity). Peruvian bark will help fight the effects of dehydration. Ask your vet for advice.

COST

If your cat has a severe case of cat flu she may have to be hospitalized and spend some time in the care of the veterinary practice. Costs can therefore be high.

Flu in cats is not uncommon, and in houses where more than one cat lives, and particularly in catteries, can soon spread to other cats. In general, the mortality rate in cats infected by cat flu is low.

Symptoms

Vary from one cat to another, but may include loss of appetite, fever, sneezing, depression, inflamed or reddened eyes, discharge from the nose, occasional coughing and ulcers on the tongue.

Underlying causes

There are two main causes, both of which are viruses. One of these is known as feline rhinotracheitis, the other as feline herpes virus. Transmission is from one affected cat to another cat in aerosol droplets from the sneezes of the infected cat(s). Unfortunately, some cats are carriers, and although they do not show any signs of the condition they can still pass cat flu to another cat.

Owner action

Any cat showing signs of cat flu should be isolated as soon as the symptoms are noticed. The incubation period is between two and ten days, but even after successful treatment, many cats which recover will still be carriers of the virus. In such cases, it is best if the affected cats are never allowed to come into contact with another cat.

Vaccinations – both injected and given via the cat's nose – can provide some protection. Your vet will advise you.

Treatment

There are two parts to treatment. The first is to nurse the cat to get her eating and drinking again, and the second is to administer drugs to alleviate her suffering. Antibiotics

DIAGNOSING CAT FLU

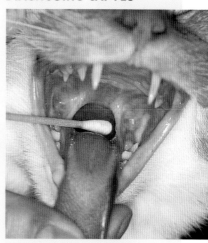

The vet will carry out a physical examination, and may take swabs from the cat's throat, which will be sent for laboratory analysis.

and mucolytics (these help clear the mucus from your cat's respiratory system) may be prescribed. Vaccination can provide some protection against cat flu.

RELATED CONDITIONS WHICH MAY PRODUCE SIMILAR SIGNS

Rhinitis (see p.10), conjunctivitis (see p.49) and bronchitis (see p.09).

Pyothorax
(Exudative pleurisy)

The accumulation of purulent material (pus) in the cat's thorax.

Symptoms
May include breathing difficulties, weight loss, increased breathing rate, fever and depression.

Underlying causes
Infection caused by a subcutaneous abscess (one under the skin), or alternatively a lung infection.

DIAGNOSING PYOTHORAX

Your vet will carry out a thorough physical examination of your cat, followed by X-ray examinations and laboratory analysis of a sample of fluid from the cat's chest.

Owner action
While you are awaiting veterinary treatment, if your cat is having severe breathing problems, place her in a steamy bathroom, and remain with her to keep her calm. The steam will help with the cat's breathing.

Treatment
Treatment will consist of finding and treating the underlying cause of the problem, although in severe cases where the cat has difficulties in breathing, the vet will give this priority. Any fluid build-up on the cat's lungs will be drained, and this will probably involve the cat being hospitalized at the veterinary practice.

RELATED CONDITIONS WHICH MAY PRODUCE SIMILAR SYMPTOMS

Pneumonia (see p.13) and chronic bronchial disease. (see p.09). ⓘ

Placing a cat in a steamy bathroom will help relieve the symptoms of pyothorax.

◐ COST
Likely to be quite high, due to the intensive treatment necessary.

Pneumonia

Inflammation of the tissue inside the cat's lungs.

Symptoms
Include incessant coughing, coughing up quite large amounts of phlegm and mucus, difficulty in breathing, reluctance to take exercise or even move at all, fever, lethargy and lack of interest in food. A cat affected by pneumonia will typically stand with her front legs spread and head lowered, often coughing, but desperate to take in more air.

Underlying causes
Pneumonia can be caused by a bacterial or a viral infection, but it can also be caused by the inhalation of food or vomit, smoke or even chemicals and, in these cases, the affected cat is highly likely to suffer from secondary bacterial pneumonia.

Owner action
Keep your cat calm while veterinary treatment is sought.

Treatment
As many body fluids are lost in the increased respiratory secretions in an affected cat, intravenous fluid therapy may be required. The vet may hospitalize your cat, and administer special drugs designed to expand the cat's airways, helping her to breathe more easily.

Where the pneumonia is caused by inhalation or aspiration, it is almost impossible for a vet to remove the foreign substances, and it is highly unlikely that the cat will make a full recovery. She will often be afflicted with a cough for the rest of her life.

RELATED CONDITIONS WHICH MAY PRODUCE SIMILAR SYMPTOMS

Cat flu (see p.11).

DIAGNOSING PNEUMONIA

The vet will use a stethoscope to detect abnormal noises from the affected cat's lungs, although x-ray examination is needed to confirm a diagnosis of pneumonia. Blood tests from an affected cat will show higher than normal numbers of white blood cells, and often the vet will take a sample of fluid and mucus from the respiratory system in order to pinpoint the exact infection responsible. This will help decide the most effective antibiotic or anti-fungal to use in each case.

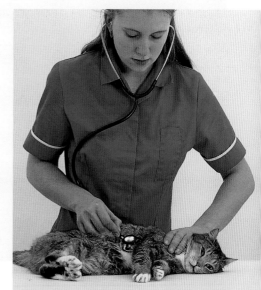

The circulatory system

The circulatory system is a series of tubes, running throughout the cat's body, through which blood circulates. The blood is driven through this system by the heart, a four-chambered, double pump in the centre of the thoracic cavity.

Blood serves many functions, including:

- **transport of oxygen to the tissues;**
- **transport of carbon dioxide away from the tissues;**
- **transport of water to the tissues;**
- **thermo-regulation;**
- **assistance in the maintenance of the correct pH in the tissues (pH is the measure of acidity (low pH) or alkalinity (high pH) – a pH of 7 is neutral);**
- **transport of waste away from the tissues;**
- **transport of food to the tissues;**
- **blood-clotting to stop haemorrhaging;**
- **transport of hormones throughout the body;**
- **transport of enzymes throughout the body; and**
- **transport of antitoxins and antibodies throughout the body (to protect against infection).**

The red colour of blood is due to the oxygen-rich haemoglobin – a protein containing iron – carried on the red blood cells. The white blood cells have the main task of protecting the body from infection. The other type of cells carried in the blood are the platelets, which help clot the blood, protecting against haemorrhage. Vitamin K is vital for this clotting, and certain rodent poisons (such as Warfarin) are designed to destroy vitamin K, thereby preventing blood clotting.

There are two parts to the circulatory system – the pulmonary and the systemic. The pulmonary circulation moves deoxygenated blood from the heart to the lungs, where carbon dioxide is expelled from the body and oxygen is taken in. This oxygenated blood is returned to the heart, from where the systemic circulation takes it to tissue and organs around the body and returns deoxygenated blood to the heart.

Blood is carried away from the heart in large blood vessels called arteries that have thick, muscular walls. Within the organs, the arteries get smaller, and are known as arterioles, and within the tissues of these organs, the arterioles become even smaller, and are then known as capillaries. These blood vessels are very thin-walled, to allow exchange of gases.

Blood is carried to the heart in large, thin-walled blood vessels called veins. When such a vessel occurs within the tissue, to receive blood from the capillary bed, it is much smaller, and is known as a venule. Blood within veins is at much lower pressure than that within arteries.

The brain, the heart and the kidneys have a system of 'end arteries', capillaries that branch throughout the three organs, but do not join with one another. It is thought that these end arteries offer protection against sudden drops in blood pressure, as would occur after severe blood loss. At times of such loss, the cat's body will divert blood to these vital organs – as the other body organs are able to survive a period of restricted blood flow without suffering damage. If an end artery becomes blocked (for example with a blood clot), blood flow is completely cut off, and the tissue will die. In the normal capillary bed, where a vessel becomes blocked, there are still many more routes through which blood can reach the tissues.

Closely allied to the circulatory system is the lymphatic system, which carries the excess tissue fluid in the body, known as lymph.

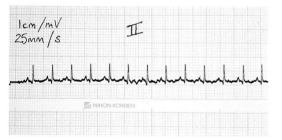

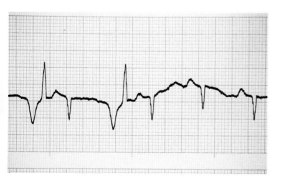

Heart problems

Heart disease is not a very common problem in cats, but where it does occur it may lead to heart failure unless the problem is treated correctly. If the movement of blood through the heart is decreased for any reason, the cat's blood pressure will increase, and there may also be a build-up of fluid in the cat's lungs or abdomen. This can lead to congestive heart failure, depending which side of the heart has the problem. To help understand the potential problems, it is necessary to look closer at the heart and the way in which it should function.

The heart is a four-chambered, double pump in the centre of the thoracic cavity. Under normal circumstances, blood enters the heart's right atrium (top chamber) via the vena cava (a large vein), and is then pumped into the right ventricle (lower chamber), before being pumped via the pulmonary artery to the cat's lungs. Blood returning from the lungs enters the heart's left atrium via the pulmonary vein, and is then pumped into the left ventricle, from where it leaves, via the aorta (a large artery), to begin its journey around the cat's body.

The atria and ventricles are separated by valves (atrio-ventricular valves), which prevent the blood from flowing in the wrong direction. Where one or more atrio-ventricular valves are defective or diseased, there is a back-flow of blood, and this causes 'heart murmurs'.

Your vet may use a electrocardiograph (ECG) to record the electrical activity of your cat's heart. The top print-out represents a normal ECG while the bottom print-out suggests an adnormality.

Cardiomyopathy

Disease of the heart muscle.

Symptoms

Fluid build-up in the lungs, causing the cat to get out of breath very easily. Her abdomen may become extended, and she may lose weight.

This disease can lead to the enlargement of the cat's heart. There are two possible effects of this condition; one is the thickening and abnormal enlargement of the heart muscle, and is known as hypertrophic cardiomyopathy. The other is thinning of the wall of the heart, and this is known as dilative cardiomyopathy.

Both hypertrophic cardiomyopathy and dilative cardiomyopathy affect the ability of the heart to contract properly.

Underlying causes

Very often, hereditary or congenital defects (present from birth). Kittens born with such defects rarely live more than a year.

Owner action

Keep the cat calm, and do not allow her to exert herself.

Treatment

If these problems are detected early in life, it may be possible to correct the problem by surgery, although this is only possible in a very small number of cases. Where the conditions are only detected later, they will cause heart disease.

Any cat showing difficulties breathing must be taken for urgent examination by a vet.

COST

Likely to be very high.

Cardiomyopathy is diagnosed by a vet listening to the cat's heart with a stethoscope.

DIAGNOSING CARDIOMYOPATHY

Using a stethoscope, the vet will listen for unusual (fast) heart rates, rhythms and murmurs. X-ray examinations will show any abnormality in the shape of the heart muscle.

RELATED CONDITIONS WHICH MAY PRODUCE SIMILAR SYMPTOMS

Certain diseases, for example bacterial infections that have spread to the heart, can affect the heart's function. It is also possible that a kitten could have a congenital heart defect; in other words, she may be born with a defect of the heart. Valvular stenosis (problems involving the heart's valves), septal defects (affecting the wall of the heart) and patent ductus arteriosus (defects of the vessels leaving the heart) have all been seen in kittens.

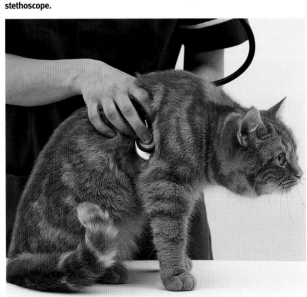

Other heart problems

Symptoms

A cat suffering from a failing heart will show certain clinical signs of the problem. Early on, these signs are liable to be subtle, so it is wise to keep a wary eye on your cat. The symptoms that an affected cat may show include breathing difficulties, coughing (especially after exercise or at night), weight loss, exercise intolerance and a distended abdomen. A cat affected by heart problems may stand with her front legs spread and head lowered, often coughing, and desperate to take in more air.

Underlying causes

There can be many causes of heart disease, some of which are congenital, such as faulty valves or a 'hole in the heart'. Heart muscle diseases and diseases of the tissues around the heart can also cause problems for the affected cat.

DIAGNOSING HEART DISEASE

Most forms of heart disease are accompanied by heart murmurs. The vet will use a stethoscope to detect these, and will be able to pinpoint the problem, from the position of the murmur and whether it occurs on the heart's relaxation phase, its contraction phase or both. The vet may also use X-rays and electrocardiograms to diagnose the exact problem.

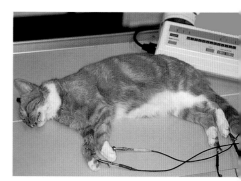

This cat is having its ECG recorded. Electrodes are placed on her paws and attached to the electrocardiograph.

Owner action

Keep the cat quiet and calm, and arrange for someone to accompany you (or preferably, to drive you) when you take your cat to be examined by the vet.

Treatment

Most cases of heart disease are not reversible, so the main aim of the vet concerned is to slow the progression of the disease. Any treatment merely makes the cat's condition easier to live with, rather than providing a cure.

To help reduce blood pressure and reduce the amount of fluid in the heart or lungs, cats with heart problems are fed on a special low-sodium diet. To reduce further the build-up of fluid, affected cats are put onto diuretics, to increase the amount of urine passed by the cat. If your cat is put on diuretics, ensure that she always has plenty of water to drink, as her thirst will increase dramatically with these drugs.

These two treatments often result in a lessening of – or even complete relief from – the coughing and discomfort associated with heart disease. If they do not, then the vet may prescribe drugs to make the work of the heart easier, by dilating the blood vessels. If even this does not work, the drug digitalis may be given. This will help slow the beat of the heart, while strengthening its contractions.

COST
The on-going nature of heart conditions means that the treatment must continue until the death of the affected cat. Consequently, the overall cost of this treatment may be quite high.

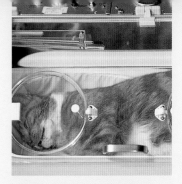

Anaemia

An overall reduction in the number of red blood cells in a cat's body, resulting in a lack of iron. This leads to the cat's cells being provided with insufficient oxygen for respiration (see p.14).

Symptoms

These include an increased breathing rate, an increased heart rate, tiredness, weakness and pale mucous membranes, such as the gums.

Underlying causes

There are many causes of anaemia. *These may include:*
● blood loss;
● cancer;
● external parasites such as fleas, ticks and lice;
● gastric ulcers;
● hookworms;
● hypothyroidism (a deficiency in the action of the thyroid gland, which produces the hormone thyroxin. This can lead to alopecia (see p.63), weight gain, fatigue and cold intolerance);
● iron deficiency;
● kidney disease (see p.38);
● liver disease (see p.93);
● poisoning; or
● vitamin B12 deficiency.

Owner action

Never attempt any home treatment of parasites unless you can and accurately identify

As the underlying cause of anaemia could be serious, you should seek veterinary advice as soon as you believe that your cat is suffering from this condition.

DIAGNOSING ANAEMIA

Diagnosis will involve the vet taking blood samples for laboratory analysis, which will be able to detect the underlying cause(s).

it. If you can, then treat in the appropriate manner; for example, treat a flea infestation with flea powder or spray. It is better not to run the risk of a mistaken identification (and hence treatment), and to have your vet confirm your identification.

Treatment

Treatment will depend upon the cause of the problem. It may be necessary for your cat to be given blood transfusions and oxygen therapy, which is the supply of pure oxygen, via a mask or an oxygen tent.

Feline infectious anaemia (FIA)

A disease which is not yet fully understood, but which gives very similar symptoms to those of severe anaemia.

Symptoms

Very similar to 'normal' anaemia (see p.18), including an increased breathing

COST

Costs will vary with types of treatment; for example, blood transfusions will increase the overall cost of the treatment.

RELATED CONDITIONS WHICH MAY PRODUCE SIMILAR SYMPTOMS

Feline infectious anaemia

URGENCY INDICATOR

It is recommended that veterinary advice is sought urgently.

Thrombosis

rate, an increased heart rate, tiredness, weakness and pale mucous membranes, such as the gums.

DIAGNOSING FIA

The vet will take blood samples for laboratory analysis.

Underlying causes
FIA is spread by fleas and ticks from one infected cat to another. It is not yet known exactly what causes this anaemia, but it is though to be the organism *Haemobartonella felis*, an endoparasite that attacks and damages the cat's red blood cells.

Owner action
Always consult your vet if you suspect that your cat may have any form of anaemia.

Treatment
Antibiotics and iron supplements will be prescribed for the anaemia, but the underlying cause may be much more difficult to tackle, and an affected cat will rarely make a full recovery, often relapsing and requiring more treatment.

RELATED CONDITIONS WHICH MAY PRODUCE SIMILAR SYMPTOMS

Anaemia (see p.18).

◉ COST
Costs may be quite high, as cats often relapse and require further treatment.

A blood clot that blocks a blood vessel.

Symptoms
A sudden onset of paralysis, often in the hind legs. Because of the lack of blood circulation, the affected legs will feel cold to the touch and be painful to the cat.

DIAGNOSING THROMBOSIS

X-ray examination may be necessary. This will reveal the actual position of the blood clot, and may also help to indicate the underlying causes of the clot.

Underlying causes
A blood clot that blocks a blood vessel. The clot is caused by the flow of blood being impeded in some way, and the clot itself further impedes the blood flow.

Owner action
Keep your cat calm and contact the vet as soon as possible.

Treatment
In very mild cases, it may be possible to treat the cat with anti-coagulants (drugs that 'thin' the blood, helping it to flow more easily) while in other cases surgery may be used to remove the clot. Unfortunately, in may cases there is no effective treatment for thrombosis, but your vet may administer analgesics (painkillers).

URGENCY INDICATOR

If a cat has a sudden onset of paralysis, veterinary treatment should be sought urgently.

COST
Probably quite high as the vet will have to spend much time carrying out examinations and the treatment may involve surgery, which is relatively expensive.

Eating and drinking

The cat's digestive system takes food and breaks it down to simple compounds which the body can then absorb, and the waste material from this process is excreted.

The digestive system starts at the mouth, where the teeth are used to hold the food and break, rip or cut it up into smaller pieces. These pieces are then manipulated by the tongue, and mixed with saliva, which moistens and lubricates the food and begins the digestive process.

Like small children, many cats also use their mouths to investigate the world around them, and this can lead to problems with the mouth and teeth. As teeth are used and abused on a daily basis, they become worn or even damaged and broken. The term periodontal diseases is used by vets to describe diseases of the teeth and gums.

Swallowed food is pushed down the pharynx (the area at the back of the throat) by muscular contractions, known as peristalsis, until it enters the stomach. In the stomach, the food is mixed with gastric juices, which break down more of the food. From the stomach, food passes into the small intestine, where more digestion occurs, and where many of the products of this digestion (amino acids, fatty acids and sugars) are absorbed. The remnants of the food pass from the small intestine into the large intestine, where water, electrolytes and water-soluble vitamins are absorbed. After all absorption has finished, the wastes remaining are passed down towards the rectum, where they are stored before being excreted.

Bad breath or halitosis

One of the most common mouth problems suffered by cats, if not the most common. Most cats show symptoms before they are three years old, and the main problem is usually gingivitis (inflammation of the gums).

Symptoms

Bad breath is often a symptom of periodontal disease (disease of the gums and/or teeth). Other signs of periodontal disease can include swollen, tender gums, loss of appetite and excessive drooling. Plaque and calculus (a build-up of minerals) on a cat's teeth can lead to heart and kidney diseases if left untreated. Yellow-brown stains on the teeth where they meet the gums are a classic symptom.

Underlying causes

Periodontal disease causes halitosis. Food sticking on or between the teeth attracts bacteria which will decay the food.

Owner action

Keep the cat's teeth in good condition. Regularly cleaning your cat's teeth can act as a preventative measure, and also as a way of inspecting the cat's teeth, and finding small problems while they can still be dealt with.

It is advisable to brush your cat's teeth regularly. Use a soft human toothbrush with a small head. *Never* use human toothpaste, as cats hate both the taste and the froth created by the paste. Brushing the cat's teeth should begin when she is a kitten, so that she gets used to the treatment. To begin with, simply use a brush dipped into warm water. Holding her mouth closed, place the brush head in the cat's cheek for a few seconds, speaking softly and reassuringly the whole time. Repeat this with the

DIAGNOSING PERIODONTAL DISEASE

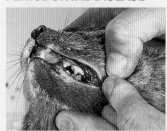

The vet will physically examine the cat's mouth. He will be looking for the underlying causes of the problem, such as tartar, plaque or even diseased tissue.

other cheek. Every day, the period should be extended until the cat is no longer concerned about the brush. At this stage, begin to move the brush in a small circle, starting with the back teeth, as these are less sensitive than the front teeth. In a couple of weeks you should be able to brush both the front and back teeth without causing the cat any concern. Then you can introduce small amounts of feline toothpaste. Rubber finger stalls may also be used instead of a toothbrush.

You should also ensure that you take your cat for a regular veterinary check-up, when her teeth will be examined.

Treatment

If your cat suffers from gingivitis, then it may be helpful to use an antiseptic spray in the cat's mouth. Ask the vet for advice on this.

Your cat's diet will greatly influence the state of her teeth. Feeding mainly soft, tinned food may adversely affect the teeth; it is much better to give at least some crunchy food (kibble or biscuit-type feed) at every mealtime.

Several manufacturers of 'dental toys' claim that they will act to clean the cat's teeth as she plays with the toy, and this is said to help keep the cat's teeth and gums in good condition.

Worn or broken teeth and abscesses

Teeth wear down through natural usage, but may also get broken. Worn teeth, on the whole, present no real problem to the cat, as any minor damage resulting from natural wear and tear is usually 'repaired' by the cat's own immune system. A broken tooth, however, will cause intense pain, suffering and distress.

Symptoms

Broken teeth are obvious when you see them, but they may be at the rear of the mouth, so be on the lookout for any abnormal behaviour which may be linked with pain in the cat's mouth. This may include difficulty eating, leading to a reluctance even to try to eat. In some cases where the cat's tooth is broken, the cat may try to eat, but cry as soon she bites into the food. This calls for a close investigation of the cat's mouth by a vet.

Abscesses result from a bacterial infection, and are pockets of pus. They may appear as soft swellings at the root of the tooth, which will sometimes burst, allowing the pus to escape. They are usually painful, and so your cat will show discomfort when she is eating.

DIAGNOSING WORN OR BROKEN TEETH

Two of you will be needed to look inside the cat's mouth. A small torch is essential. Be very careful not to get bitten, as the cat will be in pain, and may resent anyone poking around in her mouth. Your vet may use X-ray examinations to confirm a diagnosis of an abscess.

Underlying causes

Worn teeth, as well as being the result of ordinary wear and tear, may be due to excessive softness of the teeth, some malformation of the jaws, or even the direction in which the teeth are growing. Such problems may have existed since the animal was born, and simply have taken some time to show up.

Teeth can be broken as a result of fights or, more usually, in accidents (particularly road traffic accidents (RTAs). If the cat has been fed a low-calcium diet, all of her teeth and bones will be much more likely to fracture and break.

There appear to be two main causes of apical abscesses (abscesses on the root of the tooth) – damage to the tooth itself, and damage to the blood supply to the root of the tooth. Both types of damage are usually caused by the cat chewing on hard objects, such as large bones, and the cats involved are usually middle-aged to old, although this problem can afflict a cat of any age and

URGENCY INDICATOR

While not life-threatening, broken teeth are extremely painful, and should be treated as an emergency. Seek veterinary help as soon as possible, as failure to do so may result in further damage and infection. Where you suspect that your cat has an abscess, you should consult your vet urgently. As there is little that can be done for worn teeth, there is far less urgency attached to this condition, although it is always advisable to seek veterinary attention for any ailment as soon as is practical.

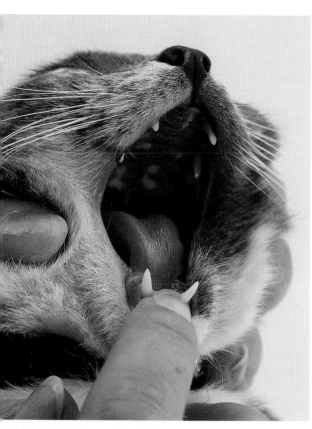

Below: To avoid worn or broken teeth you may need to change your cat's eating habits. You may also need advice on maintaining your cat's teeth.

Above: While examining your cat's mouth use a pencil torch to look for broken teeth.

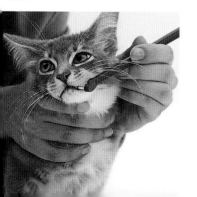

COST

Severe dental problems and injuries can be quite expensive to treat. As in humans, some dental conditions will require long and difficult sessions of surgery with your cat under a general anaesthetic.

any breed. Whatever the original cause, of the problem apical abscesses will not cure themselves, and veterinary treatment must be sought.

Owner action

Even if you cannot see any damage, if the cat exhibits symptoms of teeth problems, seek veterinary advice, as the problem may be dangerous and painful. Once the cat's condition has been properly diagnosed your vet will advise you on any change of diet that may be necessary to help maintain your cat's teeth.

Treatment

Broken teeth may be capped to seal them against bits of food or other items working their way into the damaged tooth and to prevent infection, which may cause even more problems and pain. In the case of abscesses, the source of the infection must be removed for the cat to make a complete recovery, and it is normal for the tooth to be removed, and the cat placed on a course of antibiotics. It is important that any such treatment is given regularly, and exactly as directed, and that the course is completely finished. Painkillers may also be prescribed for the cat.

In a few cases, cats suffering from dental problems may be referred to specialist dentistry vets.

RELATED CONDITIONS WHICH MAY PRODUCE SIMILAR SYMPTOMS

Many diseases of the mouth may exhibit symptoms which are very much alike. You should consult your vet if you suspect any such problems.

Diabetes mellitus

A hormonal condition in which the cat is unable to control her blood sugar levels.

Symptoms

An increase in the cat's appetite, particularly if coupled with other symptoms such as an increase in her thirst, an increase in the amount of urine passed, lethargy, weight loss and maybe cataracts (see p.50). Very often, symptoms of diabetes mellitus are seen in queens just after they have started oestrus.

Underlying causes

Diabetes mellitus or 'sugar diabetes' is caused by lack of insulin (produced by the pancreas) or an increase in blood sugar levels (hyperglycaemia). It is quite common in queens of middle age or older. The underlying problem may be quite serious, as it may indicate that the cat's pancreas is not producing enough insulin, perhaps due to an abnormality of the pancreas or through the natural ageing of the organ. It can occur in almost any cat but is most common in those over eight years of age. Due to the increased levels of progesterone (a hormone) in the blood during phantom or pseudo pregnancies (see p.81), unspayed queens are said to be more then three times more susceptible to diabetes mellitus, and obese cats of either sex are also at increased risk.

DIAGNOSING DIABETES MELLITUS

Blood and urine tests will show the levels of glucose present in the cat's system, while ultrasound and X-ray examinations will show the physical state of the cat's pancreas. 👁

URGENCY INDICATOR

If your cat shows any of the symptoms listed, seek veterinary treatment as soon as possible.

COST

Treatment for this condition is likely to be long term, as your cat may need regular insulin injections and other treatment, so the full costs in time and money will be fairly high.

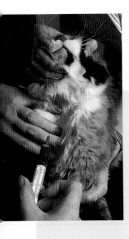

Owner action

Take any cat showing symptoms of diabetes for examination by a vet as soon as possible. Treatment will consist of an extremely strict high-fibre diet which will be prescribed by your vet. In queens, spaying will keep the cat's condition stable.

RELATED CONDITIONS WHICH MAY PRODUCE SIMILAR SYMPTOMS

Diabetes insipidus is caused by a lack of anti-diuretic hormone – ADH – (produced in the cat's pituitary glands), or the failure of the kidneys to respond to this hormone. ADH normally helps concentrate the cat's urine when she needs to conserve water. The production of ADH is increased when there is little water intake, and decreased when the cat drinks large quantities of water, thus controlling the body's water balance.

Symptoms of diabetes insipidus include polydipsia (an excessive thirst) and polyuria (production of large amounts of urine). Dependent upon which form of diabetes insipidus is present, treatment may involve the administration of ADH to the affected cat; this is administered via nasal drops.

Many of the conditions associated with diabetes mellitus are also common symptoms of other, less serious, diseases. For example an increased thirst may simply be due to your cat being fed on a dry diet. However, if your cat shows any of the symptoms described earlier, veterinary advice should be sought as soon as possible. *i*

Treatment

Treatment of the condition can be completely successful, provided that the vet is consulted before the condition becomes chronic. It will depend upon the results of all of the tests, and the type and cause of the diabetes mellitus. Possible treatments the vet may prescribe include weight loss, spaying, insulin injections, medication, a special diet and increased exercise. Whatever the treatment, it will inevitably involve you in quite a lot of work over a prolonged period of time. Typically, you will need to collect and test a sample of urine from your cat every morning to check the glucose levels, calculate the amount of insulin needed and administer it by injection, and feed your cat an extremely regulated diet at specific times. Your vet will advise you on all of these matters.

Abnormal water intake

This may be a symptom of diabetes mellitus, but it is most likely to indicate cystitis (see p.36). It may also be caused by *Dipylidium caninum,* a parasitic white tapeworm that lives in the cat's small intestine.

Symptoms

Segments of the tapeworm may be found in the feces of an infected cat. Often, the cat has an increased appetite, and may suffer irritation around her anus.

Underlying causes

Dipylidium caninum is a segmented tapeworm. The average length is 25 cm (10 in), although they can grow to twice that size. This tapeworm is transmitted via fleas.

DIAGNOSING *DIPYLIDIUM*

Physical examination of feces of the affected cat, which may be followed by laboratory analysis of the feces.

When the tapeworm segments drop off the cat, eggs are released from the segments. These eggs are then eaten by flea larvae which, when adult, attach themselves to a cat. As the cat grooms herself, fleas are ingested, and these contain immature tapeworms. The cycle repeats *ad infinitum.* The tapeworms develop inside the cat, and feed off the cat, causing her to lose weight, despite having an increased appetite.

Owner action

If you suspect that your cat has a tapeworm, ensure that you have her treated by a vet. Remember that this parasite can be passed from cat to cat, and so all cats in the household should be treated at the same time, even if they do not show any symptoms of an infestation.

Treatment

Treatment consists of prescribed worming tablets (anthelmintics).

RELATED CONDITIONS WHICH MAY PRODUCE SIMILAR SYMPTOMS

Many conditions can cause your cat to lose weight and/or have an increased appetite. These vary from cancer to insufficient or inappropriate feeding.

URGENCY INDICATOR

Not life-threatening, but treatment is best started as soon as the problem is noticed.

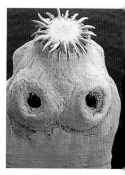

Quite often abnormal water intake is caused by *Dipylidium caninum,* a tapeworm which inhabits the small intestine.

COST

Anthelmintics are not expensive.

Toxocara cati

A parasitic white roundworm that lives in the infected cat's intestines.

Parasites cause medical problems to their host: that is, the animal on which the parasite lives. This can be by depriving the host of food, or by transmitting diseases, so treatment should be sought as soon as the problem is noticed.

Symptoms

Young kittens are more likely to become infected. The kittens may suffer from a poor coat and have diarrhoea. Typically, infected kittens have a 'pot belly' due to the build-up of gases in the intestines. Actual worms, measuring between 6 cm and 12 cm ($2\frac{1}{4}$ in and $4\frac{1}{2}$ in) long, may be seen in the kittens' feces, or may be coughed up.

Underlying causes

Kittens become infected with the parasite from their mother via the placenta while in the womb, and after birth from her milk when they suckle.

Owner action

Use de-wormers (anthelmintics) prescribed by your veterinary surgeon only. No matter how well a cat is cared for, it is impossible to prevent her from catching worms and other endoparasites, especially as animals can be infected from their mother.

⊗ COST

Anthelmintics are not expensive.

Below: **It is inevitable that kittens will inherit** *Toxocara* **infections from their mother.**

Above: **A selection of worming pills is accompanied by a record of the cat's treatment programme.**

DIAGNOSING *TOXOCARA*

Physical examination of feces of the affected cat, which may be followed by laboratory analysis of the feces.

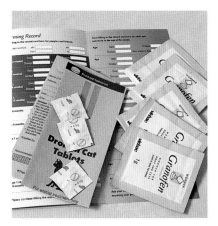

Treatment

Treatment consists of suitable prescribed anthelmintics. Queens should be treated when they are pregnant and lactating, and kittens should be treated every three weeks between the ages of four and 16 weeks. All cats should be treated every six months as a preventative measure.

RELATED CONDITIONS WHICH MAY PRODUCE SIMILAR SYMPTOMS

There are many conditions which can cause your cat to lose weight and/or have an increased appetite. These vary from cancer to insufficient or inappropriate feeding. *ⓘ*

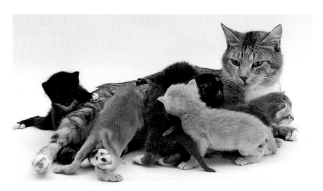

Difficulty swallowing

URGENCY INDICATOR

If you suspect your cat is suffering from any blockage of the digestive system or a problem which is preventing her from swallowing food, it is vital that immediate veterinary investigation is carried out, as a blockage can be life-threatening.

Indicates one of several possible conditions, including pharyngitis, tonsillitis or even a blockage of the digestive system. Pharyngitis is the inflammation of the pharynx, the area at the back of the throat, while tonsillitis is inflammation of the tonsils.

Symptoms
These include coughing or retching (as if the throat is blocked), loss of appetite (even though the cat is hungry) and difficulty in swallowing even water.

DIAGNOSING TONSILLITIS AND PHARYNGITIS

When inflamed, the cat's tonsils, which are not usually conspicuous, are very obvious, appearing as two very bright red lumps. X-rays will almost always be taken to confirm any diagnosis, before surgery is undertaken. If your cat is suffering from pharyngitis, the lining at the back of the throat will be red and inflamed. Inflammation of the pharynx or tonsils will block the throat itself.

COST
Depends entirely on the underlying causes and consequent treatment. If surgery is involved, costs may be high.

Underlying causes
Both pharyngitis and tonsillitis can be caused by a viral infection, a bacterial infection following damage to the area done by a foreign body, periodontal (gum) disease or other factors. Tonsillitis is particularly common in kittens and young cats, but pharyngitis may occur in any cat of any breed or age.

Owner action
Observe your cat, and note her actions. Ensure that she is given sufficient water to drink, to prevent dehydration.

Treatment
A course of antibiotics, which must be given regularly and until the course is completed, will usually clear up any infection of the tonsils or the pharynx.

Even if the vet suspects a blockage of the digestive system, they may not begin treatment immediately, preferring to observe the cat for some time first. Once the diagnosis has been confirmed, surgery may be the preferred option.

RELATED CONDITIONS WHICH MAY PRODUCE SIMILAR SYMPTOMS

Periodontal disease (see p. 21) can make it painful for the cat to eat or swallow.

A foreign body or other blockage in the digestive system is also a common cause of loss of appetite in a cat. Typically, fur collects when the cat is grooming herself, and this becomes lodged in the digestive system (see p.20). Such a blockage will cause a variety of symptoms, which may include excessive drooling, loss of appetite, regurgitation of food, vomiting, swelling of the abdomen and constipation.

Heart disease is another possible cause of loss of appetite (see p.15 and 17). In queens who have had several heats, pyometra may be a reason for loss of appetite (see p.84), while older cats may be suffering from liver failure (see p.93).

Vomiting

A symptom of another condition, not an illness itself.

Symptoms

Every reader will recognize the signs of vomiting. Vomiting is a muscular reflex action, resulting in expulsion, under force, of the contents of the cat's stomach and/or small intestine.

Underlying causes

Vomiting is often brought on by something extremely simple, such as a rapid change of diet, or motion sickness. Other causes may include heatstroke (see p.113) or other conditions that affect the chemical composition of the blood, such as diabetes mellitus (see p.24), renal failure (see p.oo), liver disease (see p.38), or a bacterial infection. A foreign body in the stomach, gastric dilation/torsion or even stomach cancer would also cause vomiting, as would a heavy load of parasitic worms, constipation (see p.32) or diarrhoea (see p.30). Fear and stress, a trauma to the head or infections may also have vomiting as a symptom.

Owner action

If your cat suddenly and repeatedly vomits, prevent her from eating or drinking anything, and contact the vet. Keep the cat where you can see her, covering the floor with newspapers or similar to keep your home clean, and note the times of vomiting, and also the consistency, colour and quantity of the vomit. By doing this, you will help the vet to find the cause of the sudden vomiting, and thereby treat the problem effectively.

Occasional vomiting is normal, and no action need be taken in such cases. However, in cases of recurring vomiting, or where large amounts of vomit are produced, or there is blood in the vomit, vet-

erinary advice should be sought. Vomiting which you consider is a result of your cat's scavenging, and which is therefore spasmodic and not severe, is best treated by starving the cat for 24 hours. During this time, it is vital that the cat is offered regular small amounts of water to drink, to help prevent dehydration. After this time, re-introduce food with small light meals, such as scrambled eggs or boiled chicken, gradually building up to her former feeding regime. If the vomiting continues, or starts again when food is re-introduced, seek veterinary advice as soon as possible.

You can help prevent some of the causes of vomiting by treating your cat on a regular basis for internal parasites (worms), discouraging her from scavenging, not making sudden changes to her diet, not feeding her prior to travelling, and not overfeeding her.

Where the vomiting is caused by hairballs (see p.35), regular grooming will reduce the risk of these. Some cats also eat grass, and this is thought to be done to make the cat vomit, presumably when she feels she has an upset stomach.

Treatment

In severe cases, it is not unusual for the affected cat to be placed on an intravenous drip to keep her hydrated. Where a foreign body is wedged in her digestive system, surgery will be needed.

Flatulence

Emission of gas from a cat's anus, often referred to as 'passing wind'.

Symptoms

A peculiar and often unpleasant smell around the cat, often combined with a characteristic noise.

Underlying causes

Flatulence may have several causes. If you feed your cat on poor quality food, she may not be able to digest it well before it passes into her large intestine, and it may begin to ferment; there may be chemical reactions within the cat's digestive system that are causing gases, or the gases may be as a result of the cat bolting her food quickly, and swallowing large amounts of air as a consequence. It may also be a symptom of serious digestive disorders, and so if the problem is persistent, it should be mentioned to the vet.

Owner action

If one particular food affects your cat by causing flatulence, change her food. It is a wise precaution to give your cat a good quality food, and avoid cheaper food of poor quality. A poor diet will have other detrimental effects on your cat, and will prevent her from becoming and staying fully fit.

Treatment

As flatulence is most often caused by diet, a change in diet will 'cure' the condition. This may mean simply avoiding some types of food or may require a complete change of diet. Such a drastic change must not be made to the cat's diet without veterinary advice.

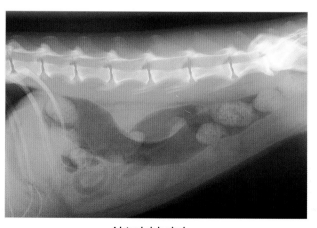

A lateral abdominal view of the build-up of colonic gas. Regular 'passing of wind' by your cat should be brought to the attention of your vet.

 HOMEOPATHIC TREATMENT:
In cases where 'rich' food is the problem, nux vomica (poison nut) may be effective. The vet will advise you.

COST
If the problem is simply diet, then the cost is likely to be low, although the cat may need to have a special 'veterinary' diet, which can work out expensive in the long term.

Diarrhoea

Like vomiting, this is a symptom of another condition and not an illness in itself.

Symptoms

Every reader will recognize the signs of diarrhoea. Greasy-looking feces and feces of different colours than usual are also classed as diarrhoea, as are small amounts of normal-looking feces that a cat passes very frequently, often having accidents around the home, despite being fully house-trained. If your cat is suffering from colitis, an inflammation of the colon (the first part of the large intestine), her feces will contain quite a lot of blood and mucus. This blood has an appearance totally different from the blood seen with internal bleeding. With internal bleeding, the blood will look dark brown and tarry, while with colitis, the blood will usually appear bright red. Another symptom of colitis is tenesmus, where the cat strains to defecate; this latter symptom is often mistaken for a symptom of constipation.

Underlying causes

Diarrhoea may simply be a symptom of over-eating, or stress. Endoparasites such as coccidia and whip worm are two of the most common causes of colitis in cats. There can, of course, be many other possible causes of diarrhoea – including foreign bodies in the digestive system and fungal infections.

Owner action

Prevent the cat from eating anything, but ensure that she is given adequate amounts of drinking water. If the diarrhoea is acute, provide the cat with a re-hydrating fluid. Contact the vet. Keep your cat where you can see her, covering the floor with newspapers or similar to keep your home clean, and note the times of her

URGENCY INDICATOR

Diarrhoea causes the cat to dehydrate, and can lead to irreparable body damage (particularly of the kidneys) and even death. In all cases of severe diarrhoea, where over-eating is definitely not the cause, you should contact the vet. If the diarrhoea persists, or if there is blood in the motions, consult the vet immediately.

◉ COST

Most cases of diarrhoea, especially those caused by simple dietary problems, will be cured at little cost. Barium meals and other such investigations will involve more veterinary care and treatment, so the cost will be considerably higher.

DIAGNOSING CAUSES OF DIARRHOEA

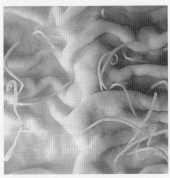

Laboratory analysis of samples of feces may be taken by the vet to ascertain the underlying cause of diarrhoea in your cat. If your cat suffers recurrent attacks of colitis, then X-rays and barium meals may be used to help find the best and most effective treatment for the condition. ◉

motions, and also the consistency, colour and quantity of the diarrhoea. By doing this, you will help the vet to find the cause of the sudden diarrhoea, and to treat the problem effectively.

The cause of diarrhoea may be a disease that can be transmitted to humans (zoonotic). Such diseases include campylobacter and salmonella, both caused by harmful bacteria. Take commonsense hygiene precautions to reduce the chance of any of these zoonotic diseases being passed on to you and your family. Always wash your hands after handling your cat, and particularly before eating. If you know that your cat has an infectious disease, you must make sure that everyone washes their hands following any contact with the affected animal.

Isolate the affected cat(s) and keep them on water and electrolytes for 24 hours, dosing with kaolin solution, available from vets, doctors and pharmacies, about every two hours. After the fast, food intake should gradually be built up again; do not put the cats straight back on their original diet, otherwise the whole problem may recur. Chicken, rabbit and fish are excellent foods for a recovering cat.

Treatment

The treatment for diarrhoea depends upon the underlying cause. If it is due to internal parasites, then anthelmintics (wormers) will be used to rid the cat of the infestation, while for infections, antibiotics will be used.

RELATED CONDITIONS WHICH MAY PRODUCE SIMILAR SYMPTOMS

Enteritis (see below). *i*

Enteritis

Inflammation of the intestines, causing diarrhoea. This is very common among young cats.

Symptoms

Diarrhoea, and signs of blood in the diarrhoea, may indicate this condition.

Underlying causes

Enteritis is very common among young cats. It can be caused by different things but often it is the bacterium *Escherichia coli*, referred to as *E. coli*. Another major cause of enteritis is *Campylobacter* bacteria; in humans, 'food poisoning' of this type is known as dysentery.

Owner action

Observe your cat's actions, and the amount,

DIAGNOSING ENTERITIS

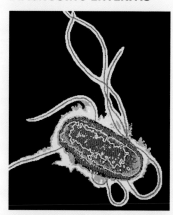

The bacterium *Escherichia coli*. In many cases of diarrhoea, the vet will want to send samples of the cat's feces for laboratory analysis, to ensure effective treatment of the problem. ◎

colour, consistency, and smell of your cat's motions. In particular, look for any signs of blood in the feces.

Treatment

Immediate treatment of enteritis a broad-spectrum antibiotic, together with regular doses of kaolin, may cure this condition. Sometimes more than one antibiotic is needed, or even two or more courses of antibiotics.

RELATED CONDITIONS WHICH MAY PRODUCE SIMILAR SYMPTOMS

All cats are potentially at risk from diarrhoea (see p.30), with young cats being more likely to suffer than adult cats. *i*

 COST

This depends on how severe the infection is.

Constipation

Failure by the cat to pass feces (or passing few and less frequently than usual). A symptom, not a disease, which may have many underlying causes. It is fairly common in elderly cats.

Symptoms

A cat producing extremely dry feces, or straining while (attempting to) defecate are all signs of constipation. Every cat and its lifestyle is different, but cats should be expected to defecate between one and four times daily.

Underlying causes

Any debilitating disease can cause constipation, as can a foreign body blocking the cat's digestive system (usually this occurs in the intestines).

Owner action

Providing your cat with a diet high in fibre and giving a good overall balanced diet will help prevent many cases of constipation.

Treatment

Where an internal blockage is the cause, the cat will need surgery. In cases linked with diet, laxatives and a change of diet may be all that is needed.

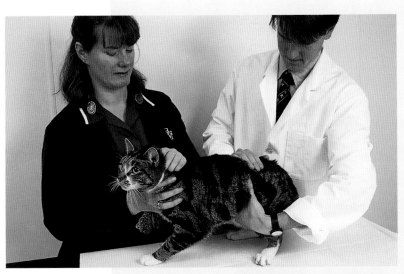

⊙ COST
If surgery is needed,
costs could be high.

DIAGNOSING CAUSES OF CONSTIPATION

A physical examination, particularly of the cat's rectum, will be necessary. In many cases, X-rays will also be taken to check that there is no physical blockage present.

Feline infectious enteritis (FIE)
(Feline panleukopenia)

A virus that attacks the white blood cells and the cat's gut.

Symptoms
These include loss of appetite, persistent vomiting and/or diarrhoea, and depression.

DIAGNOSING FELINE INFECTIOUS ENTERITIS

The vet will send a sample of blood for laboratory analysis.

Underlying causes
A widespread and highly infectious viral disease, which is passed from one infected cat to another by direct or indirect contact.

Owner action
This disease is highly infectious, so isolate any infected cats. To guard against this life-threatening disease, ensure that your cat is vaccinated, and receives regular boosters.

Treatment
There is no real treatment for FIE, but special care and intensive nursing may help alleviate the symptoms.

FIE is a very serious condition. If your cat shows any of the sypmtoms mentioned above, including, vomiting, you should seek veterinary treatment immediately.

COST
Due to the chronic nature of this disease, and the intensive care that may be necessary, treatment costs may be high.

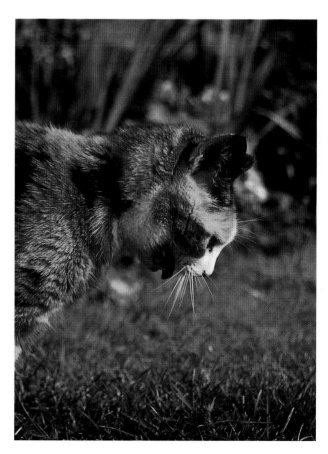

Feline infectious peritonitis (FIP)

Caused by a virus that affects cat under about three years of age. It is known to spread rapidly among cats, and so is particularly dangerous in households where there is more than one cat.

Symptoms
These include loss of appetite, a swollen abdomen, loss of weight, breathing problems and a fever.

Underlying causes
A virus, feline coronavirus, which is passed from one infected cat to another by direct or indirect contact.

Owner action
Isolate infected cats and seek urgent veterinary advice.

Treatment
There is no treatment for FIP, and most cats will die as a direct result of this infection. It may be advisable to have your cat put to sleep; your vet will help you to make this decision.

DIAGNOSING FELINE INFECTIOUS PERITONITIS

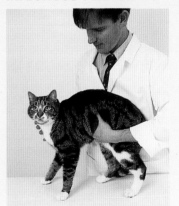

The vet will send a sample of blood for laboratory analysis.

 COST
As stated earlier, there is no specific treatment for this condition.

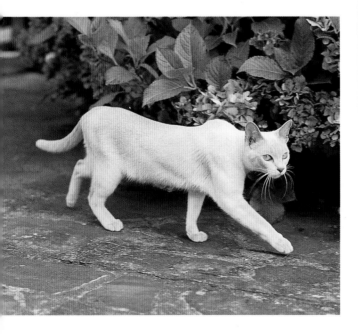

The loss of appetite and subsequent weight loss is one of the symptoms of this life-threatening virus.

Hairballs

The accumulation of hair in a cat's digestive system, as a direct result of the cat grooming herself.

Symptoms
If the hairball is in the stomach, the cat will vomit it up. If it is further down the digestive system, and causing a blockage, the cat may have a decreased appetite, constipation and suffer from general lethargy.

DIAGNOSING HAIRBALLS

If there is a blockage in the intestine, a physical examination, together with X-ray examinations, will reveal where the blockage is.

Underlying causes
As cats groom themselves, small amounts of hair are ingested. Normally, the hair passes through the digestive system and out in the feces. Sometimes, however, the amount of hair can cause a problem, particularly in long-haired breeds, and also at times of moult (usually spring and autumn). At such times, the hair accumulates in the cat's stomach. This leads to a solid mass, which then rubs against the lining of the stomach, and this irritation causes the cat to vomit.

Owner action
Regularly grooming your cat, particularly at times of moult, will reduce the risk of hairballs causing problems.

Treatment
If your cat has a mild blockage, liquid paraffin may help the passage of the hairball. In severe cases, surgery may be needed.

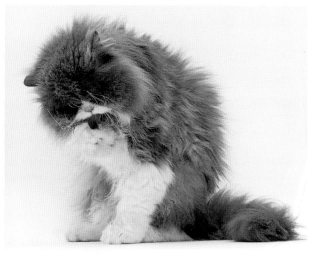

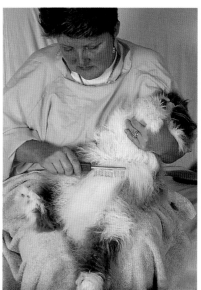

Above: **While grooming themselves cats ingest fur which causes hairballs to form in the digestive system.**

Right: **To reduce the creation of hairballs, groom your cat regularly.**

Cystitis

Inflammation of the bladder. It can affect both toms and queens.

Symptoms
These include urinating more frequently than usual, but often passing quite small amounts of urine, or the animal showing severe discomfort when urinating. The urine may be blood-stained or foul-smelling and the consistency may be thicker than normal. Cystitis is far more common in female cats (including spayed females) than in males.

DIAGNOSING CYSTITIS
A number of different bacteria may be the cause of cystitis, so a sample of urine from the affected cat will be required for the vet to diagnose and treat the condition accurately.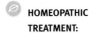

Underlying causes
Most cases of cystitis are caused by a bacterial infection of the bladder from the genitals. Sometimes the cause is the presence of bladder stones.

Owner action
Ensure that the cat has plenty of clean drinking water.

Treatment
In straightforward cases of cystitis, the cat is usually treated with a course of antibiotics. The antibiotics must be given regularly, as directed by the vet, and the course must be finished for a full recovery.

COST
Antibiotics are not expensive.

HOMEOPATHIC TREATMENT:
Depending on the underlying causes of the condition, nux vomica, chimaphila or cantharis may be effective in the treatment of cystitis. Your vet will advise you further.

URGENCY INDICATOR

Cystitis is not life-threatening, although it is often extremely distressing and painful for the affected animal. Veterinary treatment should therefore be sought as soon as possible.

Antibiotics must be given regularly, or they may not work. Your vet will show you the best way to administer pills.

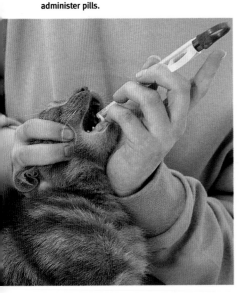

RELATED CONDITIONS WHICH MAY PRODUCE SIMILAR SYMPTOMS

Diabetes mellitus (see p.24) is another possible cause of frequent urination, as is trauma of the bladder (usually caused in an RTA, [road traffic accident], or similar accident) and bladder 'stones'.

A cat may develop stones in her urinary system (usually but not always in the bladder). These stones are known as uroliths, and the condition as urolithiasis (see p.76).

Urinary incontinence

The inability to control urination.

Symptoms

The cat will have accidents, particularly at night time. She will not have urinated deliberately, but because of her condition, the urine will dribble out when she is lying down.

DIAGNOSING URINARY INCONTINENCE

Laboratory analysis of the affected cat's urine, X-rays and ultrasound may all be required to get a full and accurate diagnosis of the condition.

Underlying causes

There are many possible cause of urinary incontinence, which may include faulty urethral valves, congenital defects of the cat's urinary system, urolithiasis (see p.76), cancer (see p.99) or prostate problems (in male cats – see p.77). This problem is seen particularly in older queens.

Owner action

When taking your cat for veterinary examination, take along a fresh sample of the affected cat's urine.

It is unfair to punish or reproach a cat for incontinence. Instead, you should ensure that she has a litter tray handy in which to relieve herself during the night, and that she is encouraged to use this before the family go to bed. Her own bed is likely to become soiled, so her bedding must be changed and cleaned at regular and frequent intervals, preferably daily.

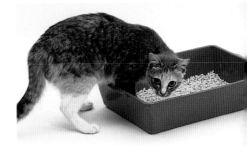

Leave your cat's litter tray near so she can relieve herself in the night.

Treatment

Surgery may be needed to treat faulty urethral valves, congenital defects of the cat's urinary system, urolithiasis (see p.76), cancer (see p.99) or prostate problems (in male cats see p.77), while drug therapy may be used to improve the effectiveness of the urethra in sealing the flow of urine.

HOMEOPATHIC TREATMENT:

Depending on the underlying cause of the problem, low-potency oestrogen, causticum, gelsemium, turnera and ustilago can be effective. Consult your vet for advice.

COST

This will vary enormously, depending on the underlying cause(s) of the condition.

Renal failure

Failure of the kidneys. Waste products from digesting protein are removed from the cat's body by the kidneys; these two organs also regulate the body's water levels, and filter the blood to maintain the levels of various chemicals in the body fluids. They pass the waste products along to the bladder through the nephrons in the form of urine. The nephrons are parts of the kidneys which remove various substances such as urea, uric acid and excess sodium from the blood.

Symptoms
They include a seemingly insatiable thirst, the passing of large amounts of urine either in one go or at very frequent intervals, vomiting, diarrhoea, loss of appetite, weight loss, halitosis and anaemia.

Underlying causes
For various reasons, including infections and physical damage, the nephrons may fail to do their job properly, and this will lead to chronic renal failure. This is an extremely serious and usually irreversible condition with a very poor chance of recovery. The condition rarely occurs in cats under the age of five years.

Owner action
Any cat showing signs of renal failure should immediately be taken for veterinary examination.

Treatment
Treatment of an affected cat may include a period of intensive care, during which the cat will have fluids administered via an intravenous drip, a special diet, coupled with a restful lifestyle and a prescribed course of medication. A cat suffering from renal failure will die, and you may choose to have your cat put to sleep.

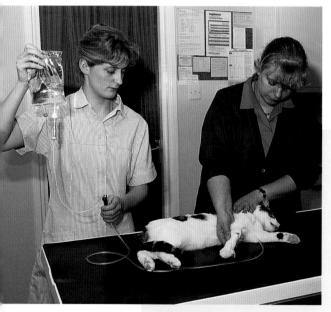

DIAGNOSING RENAL FAILURE

The vet will arrange laboratory analysis of urine, X-rays and ultrasound examinations. These tests will look for signs that the kidneys are not working, that is the nephrons are not removing urea, uric acid and sodium from the blood plasma.

◷ COST
Due to the long-term nature of the intensive treatment required, veterinary costs will be high.

Anal gland problems

The cat has two anal sacs, just below the anus; one is at 8 o'clock and the other at 4 o'clock. They secrete an oily, light brown liquid, that is expressed via two tubes as feces pass through the anus. It is thought that this liquid, which smells very bad to humans, is used as a means of recognition between individual cats, and amounts are deposited along with every piece of feces passed by the cat. These sacs can become infected. This condition is far more common in dogs than it is in cats.

Symptoms
In an effort to relieve her discomfort, an affected cat may take to licking the area around the anus, and this can cause further problems. A cat who licks at her infected anal glands will spread the infection to her mouth or throat, and this may lead to tonsillitis or pharyngitis. Where a cat is overweight, she may not be able to get to her anal glands, and so will be seen to nibble and lick at her flanks as she attempts to relieve the pain around her anus.

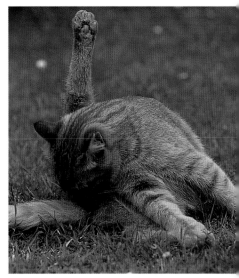

A cat which spends much time licking around its anus may be suffering from problems with its anal sac. A trip to the vet is called for.

DIAGNOSING ANAL GLAND PROBLEMS

The vet will carry out a physical examination of the cat's rectum.

Underlying causes
When the liquid in the anal sacs becomes thicker, which may be due to an infection, it may become more difficult for the liquid to be expressed, and this leads to a condition known as overfilling. If the cat starts producing the liquid at a faster rate, or the muscle tone around the anus alters, this can also lead to overfilling. The liquid in the overfilled sac then becomes impacted, and the sacs may become infected, causing the cat distress and pain.

Owner action
If your cat shows any of the symptoms listed above, she should be taken for examination by the vet; if there is a discharge from the anal sacs she should be taken as soon as possible.

Treatment
If the problem is found to be overfilled anal sacs, the vet will empty them, which will ease the cat's discomfort. If the sacs are infected, then the cat may need to be given a general anaesthetic, and have her sacs flushed out. Antibiotics will be given to a cat with infected anal sacs.

Movement

Movement (or locomotion) in cats is brought about by the musculoskeletal system. This is made up of muscles, bones, ligaments, cartilage, tendons (tough bands made from fibres which attach muscle to bones) and other supportive structures. The system also supports and protects the animal's vital organs.

In the cat, the forelimb is joined to the trunk of the animal not by a socket joint, but by muscles alone. This arrangement is ideal for an animal such as the cat, which has to run to live, as it gives a form of shock absorber, rather than the jarring which would result from a bony attachment. The hind limbs produce the main propulsion for the cat, so they are joined by a rigid bone called the pelvic girdle. Unlike dogs, cats have a rudimentary collar bone.

Normally, all of the cat's bones, muscles, ligaments, cartilage, tendons and other supportive structures work well together to keep the cat mobile. However, accidents can happen, and certain diseases will interfere with the workings of the musculoskeletal system. Any disorders, problems or ailments concerning the musculoskeletal system are likely to be extremely painful and disabling for the cat.

Lameness

A cat is lame if she is incapable of normal locomotion, or she moves with a gait that is not normal.

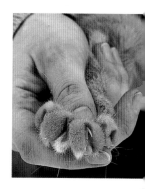

In any case of lameness, the cat's feet should be examined for cuts, splinters or thorns.

Symptoms
The cat may 'favour' a leg, or limp; in severe cases, the cat may not put the foot to the floor, or even walk at all.

Underlying causes
Lameness may be caused by a variety of conditions but, in general, it is a symptom of pain in a limb or supporting tissues. Lameness may also be caused by deformities such as short limbs, or by the abnormal shortening of the muscles of the limbs.

Some causes of lameness are easily corrected, such as splinters in a paw, or a broken claw, while others are caused simply by parts wearing out in an older cat.

DIAGNOSING CAUSES OF LAMENESS

Physical examination of the affected feet or legs should be undertaken. The vet may need to use X-rays and other examinations to find the cause of any lameness.

Owner action
The first place to look for the cause of sudden mild lameness is the cat's paw. Examine it carefully for any obvious injury such as a cut or graze, a foreign body, balled fur, or a piece of grit; this is likely to be in one of the pads under the foot. If the injury is a small foreign body, such as a grass seed, it should be carefully removed with a pair of tweezers. The wound should then be cleaned with saline solution, and a little antiseptic ointment applied.

With long-haired cats, the hair between the toes can ball up and make walking very uncomfortable. Any such fur should be gently trimmed off, using round-ended scissors to avoid stabbing the cat's foot if she moves. It is very useful to have someone to help you do this.

During winter, your cat may pick up pieces of salt grit, which will have been spread on the road to help reduce the effects of frost, ice and snow. This grit has a nasty habit of getting into a cat's feet, making walking extremely painful for the cat. If there is evidence of salt grit in the feet, wash the affected feet in warm water. After washing, inspect the feet again, and apply antiseptic ointment to any area where the skin is inflamed or broken.

During the summer months, grass seeds are a potential problem for cats, particularly active cats who spend much time in grassed fields and other areas. Grass seeds are particularly dangerous because their shape helps them to 'worm' their way into the skin, but makes extraction very difficult indeed.

Treatment
Where the lameness is only mild, but has suddenly appeared, it is likely that the problem is simple, and therefore easy to cure. Where the cat is suffering from acute lameness, the treatment will depend entirely on the underlying causes.

If a grass seed has entered the cat's skin, and it is not found, surgery may be necessary to remove it.

Fractures

Damage to bones caused by direct or indirect pressure. The bones may bend, split, crack, shatter or actually break. Where the bone is broken and pierces the skin, this is known as an open or compound fracture. Where there is one break that does not pierce the skin, it is a closed or simple fracture. Where a bone is broken into several pieces, the condition is known as a comminuted fracture. Any bones in the cat's body may fracture, although the most common fractures are those of the feet and legs.

Symptoms

Painful movement of the limb, tenderness, swelling, loss of control of the limb, deformity of the limb, unnatural movement of the limb, and crepitus (the sensation or, in very bad cases, the sound of the two ends of the bones grinding on each other).

DIAGNOSING FRACTURES

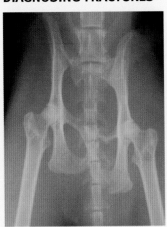

X-ray examination is almost always used to confirm fractures and also to discover the exact nature and extent of the fracture.

If you suspect that your cat has a broken bone, veterinary treatment should be sought immediately. Fractures may cause other complications, particularly if left untreated. In RTAs, although the most obvious injury may be a fracture, there could be other, potentially life-threatening, injuries as well.

🕐 **COST**
Complicated and multiple fractures may require more than one operation to carry out all of the work, adding to the overall cost.

Underlying causes

Most fractures are caused by falls, road traffic accidents (RTAs), or where the cat has been kicked by a horse or similar animal. Kittens' bones are rather flexible, and can withstand quite major trauma without fracturing. However, where a cat has been fed a calcium-poor diet and the bones have not had the opportunity to grow strong, they will be very susceptible to fractures.

Owner action

Keep the cat quiet, and steady and support the injured limb, immobilizing it with bandages and splints if necessary, to prevent it moving and causing greater damage. Raising the limb will help reduce discomfort and swelling (by reducing the blood flow). Veterinary attention should be sought for every (suspected) fracture.

Treatment

Treatment depends on the extent and position of the fracture, but the aim is to allow the bone to mend itself. The first part of this process is to get the two broken ends to join, and then to prevent them from moving until the repair is healed. The most common method of holding the broken pieces of bone in place is by the use of casts and splints. In this method, once the broken ends have been manipulated back into position, a rigid splint and/or plaster cast will be applied.

Surgery may be required to screw metal plates on to the pieces of bone, or in some cases just screws are used to keep the bone in place. One method that is common where long bones are involved, such as the main leg bones, is the use of long metal pins. Once the broken parts have been manipulated back into place, the pins are inserted down the centre of the bone, through the bone marrow. Wire is used to

Dislocation

prevent any movement or twisting of the separate parts of the bone.

While many cats will be allowed home within a few hours or days of surgery to repair fractures, others may have to spend a lot longer at the veterinary practice to ensure maximum care and effective treatment. Once your cat is back at home, you will probably need to administer prescribed painkillers and antibiotics (to treat any infection), and perhaps to change dressings. It is important that you follow carefully the instructions that the vet gives you regarding medicines, feeding and movement. You will probably need to take the cat back to the vet for regular check-ups and, eventually, for the removal of casts, splints, screws or plates.

Whichever methods are used to repair fractures, the cat's rate of recovery will vary depending on several factors. Young cats are likely to recover more quickly than older cats, bones that have fractured into only two pieces will mend quicker than those with more breaks, while any infection will lengthen the whole process, regardless of other factors involved.

The displacement of a bone from its joint.

Symptoms
Pain and swelling, loss of movement and paralysis. These symptoms are often accompanied by shock (see p.115).

Underlying causes
Causes of dislocation can include bad falls, road traffic accidents (RTAs), fights, and even normal leaping and jumping.

Owner action
If you suspect that your cat is suffering from a dislocation of a joint, you should keep the cat still and calm, and seek immediate veterinary attention.

Treatment
Treatment will usually consist of literally popping the joint back into its proper place. Most cats are sedated or anaesthetized during the procedure. Painkillers will probably be prescribed. Rest leading to steady, easy exercise will help your cat to make a complete recovery.

In all cases of injury involving suspected dislocations of joints, urgent veterinary treatment should be sought for the injured cat.

RELATED CONDITIONS WHICH MAY PRODUCE SIMILAR SYMPTOMS

Many diseases of the mouth may exhibit symptoms which are very much alike. You should consult your vet if you suspect any such problems. ⓘ

DIAGNOSING DISLOCATIONS

X-ray and physical examinations will help the vet to diagnose the problem correctly.

RELATED CONDITIONS WHICH MAY PRODUCE SIMILAR SYMPTOMS

Fractures (see p.42) and paralysis (see p.46).

🕒 **COST**
Unlikely to be too high in simple cases of dislocation of a joint, although any complications arising from the injury will add to the cost. Complications can include damaged ligaments, or the joint may need pinning.

Arthritis

Inflammation of the joints. There are two forms of arthritis that may affect cats – osteoarthritis and traumatic arthritis.

Symptoms

Swollen joints, difficulty in walking, lameness.

Underlying causes

Osteoarthritis may be a condition in itself, or a result of other conditions. It is a progressive and painful disease which will seriously affect the quality of life of the affected cat. It may affect one or more joints, and the seriousness of the condition will depend on which joints are affected, and the general health of the cat. Osteoarthritis is not nearly as common in cats as it is in dogs. Overweight cats are more prone to osteoarthritis.

Traumatic arthritis is caused as a direct result of an injury to the joint, for example the result of a road traffic accident (RTA) or a sprain while exercising.

Owner action

Your vet will advise you as to what action you should take, as this will depend on the underlying causes and treatment being given.

Treatment

The treatment for arthritis may include anti-inflammatory drugs and painkillers, and in some cases surgery may be needed.

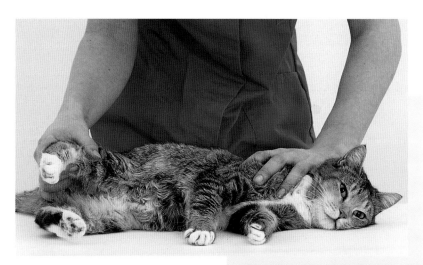

COST

In established osteoarthritis, the ongoing treatment could prove to be expensive.

DIAGNOSING ARTHRITIS

Physical examination and observation of the cat's movement will give the vet an indication of the problem. X-ray examination and analysis of samples of fluid taken from the affected joint(s) will often be necessary.

Spondylosis

A degenerative disease of the bones in the spine (vertebral column).

Any cat showing symptoms of lameness should be taken for veterinary examination as soon as possible.

Symptoms
They include dragging of the feet and lack of co-ordination.

Underlying causes
Affected cats are usually between eight and 12 months old, although spondylosis may also occur as a consequence of wear and tear, and so may be seen in elderly cats. This condition is uncommon in cats.

Owner action
Keep the cat comfortable, and seek veterinary advice.

Treatment
There is no cure for spondylosis; veterinary treatment will consist of trying to alleviate the pain and discomfort associated with the condition.

 COST

As there is no treatment for this disease, the costs will be for painkillers and other drugs to help improve your cat's quality of life.

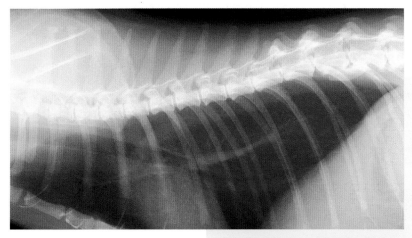

DIAGNOSING SPONDYLOSIS

The vet will confirm the diagnosis by X-ray examination (radiography).

Paralysis

Inability to move a limb or part of the body, or loss of feeling in part(s) of the body.

Symptoms

Paralysis is a symptom of disruption of the nervous system. Affected muscles cannot work normally, and internal organs may be affected. The affected cat may not be able to move the affected limb, or may drag it.

DIAGNOSING CAUSES OF PARALYSIS

X-ray and ultrasound examinations may be used to determine the underlying cause of the paralysis.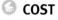

Underlying causes

Paralysis can be caused by any injury or trauma to the cat's brain, nerves or spine; road traffic accidents are a major cause of such injuries. Infectious diseases and infections may also bring on paralysis.

Owner action

Keep the cat calm and prevent any attempts at movement until a vet has carried out a thorough examination.

Treatment

The effectiveness of therapy will depend on the extent of the nervous injury and the time elapsed between the injury and the beginning of therapy. Therapy will vary with the type of paralysis, but may involve drugs, hydrotherapy or physiotherapy. In some cases, a combination of two or more therapies may be required.

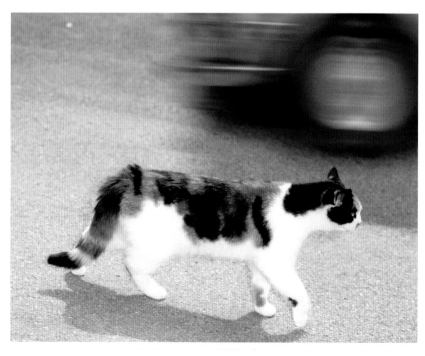

COST

There are many underlying causes of paralysis, so the treatment costs could be quite high.

Poor exercise tolerance

With most cats, it is often difficult to provide the cat with enough exercise, but sometimes, a normally active cat will develop problems that make exercise difficult for her.

Symptoms
Pain and discomfort during what should be normal exercise.

Underlying causes
Often poor tolerance to exercise is a direct result of inflammation of the joints (arthritis – see p.44). Where a muscle is diseased (for example with a bacterial infection) this is referred to as myopathy, and where a muscle is inflamed, this is referred to as myositis.

Owner action
Be very careful with regard to administering painkillers for sprains etc., unless under veterinary instruction. Painkillers can easily lull a cat into a false sense of security, causing it to use injured joints which will result in more severe damage.

Treatment
In cases of mild myopathy, for example, where your cat develops a slight limp for 24–36 hours, simply resting her will probably relieve the problem (sometimes it will be necessary to confine her to a carry box or similar), although if the limp persists beyond this time, veterinary advice and treatment should be sought.

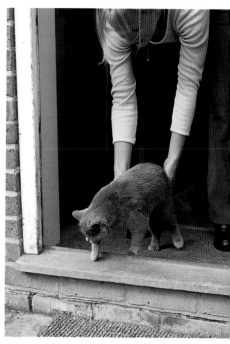

Inflammation of the joints may be the reason a usually active cat appears lacklustre.

DIAGNOSING CAUSES OF POOR EXERCISE TOLERANCE

Physical and X-ray examinations.

RELATED CONDITIONS WHICH MAY PRODUCE SIMILAR SYMPTOMS

Lameness (see p.41), paralysis (see p.46) and arthritis (see p.44).

 COST
Sprains will cost very little in treatment costs.

Eye conditions

The eyeball or globe consists of three layers:

- **the outer layer, which includes the cornea;**
- **the middle layer, which contains the iris; and**
- **the inner layer, the retina.**

The transparent part of the eyeball, or cornea, allows the cat to see out. Through this, you can see the iris and the pupil. The middle layer contains the ligament which holds the lens. This lens focuses light on the retina, which contains light-sensitive cells, called rods and cones. Cones are responsible for colour vision. Within the retina lies the optic nerve, through which the eye sends signals to the brain.

The eye is a very complex and vital organ. Any injury or damage to or abnormality of the eye should be referred to a vet immediately. Failure to act quickly may result in the cat suffering permanent damage to the eye or even total blindness.

Some eye conditions are hereditary, and some breeds are more prone to certain eye problems than others. Long-haired breeds are prone to blocked tear ducts; Abyssinian and Siamese cats have inherited eye problems and may squint a lot. This squinting is due to the fact that they suffer from double vision and reduced binocular vision (binocular vision is seeing with both the eyes at the same time). If you are purchasing a pedigree cat, then you should check with the breeders to ensure that the kitten's parents have both been screened for any hereditary eye problems. Many responsible breeders are breeding out these problems by using selective breeding techniques (only breeding from animals that do not have these problems) .

WARNING: NEVER TRY TO TREAT ANY EYE PROBLEMS YOURSELF: ALWAYS SEEK VETERINARY ADVICE.

Conjunctivitis

HOMEOPATHIC TREATMENT:
The homeopathic treatment of eye conditions is well established, and enjoys a high degree of success. Many remedies can be used on conjunctivitis, including euphrasia, aconite, pulsatilla and sanicula. Ask your vet for advice.

COST
Not high in mild cases. If left, the condition will worsen, and the cost of treatment will increase.

Inflammation of the membrane on the inner eyelids and over the eyeball, or the third eyelid (the nictitating membrane). This may be acute (appears rapidly) or chronic (appears slowly, lasts a long time and is resistant to treatment). It may affect one or both eyes, and is the major cause of reddened eyes. Even relatively mild cases of conjunctivitis can lead to the affected cat injuring her eye when scratching at the irritation. Many of the underlying causes of conjunctivitis can be very dangerous for the affected cat.

Symptoms
Include reddened eyes, a thick discharge from the corner of one or both eyes, increased blinking, 'crying' (increased tear production), half-closed eyes, constant scratching around the eyes, or rubbing of the face on hard objects or along the floor.

DIAGNOSING CONJUNCTIVITIS

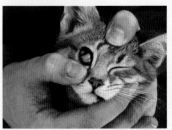

The vet will remove any discharge from around the eye and then carefully examine the cat's eyes using an ophthalmoscope. The eyeball surface will be examined in more detail. Samples may be taken from the cat's eye(s) for laboratory analysis, to help find the cause of the problem.

Underlying causes
Conjunctivitis can be caused by allergies, infections (bacterial, fungal or viral) such as feline respiratory disease (see p.11) or physical damage (for example, from thorns, grass seeds or other foreign bodies lodged in the eye).

Owner action
Look for any reddening of the cat's eyes. If you think there is a foreign body in the eye, do not try to remove it with a solid object such as a finger, cotton bud or tweezers (forceps), as you may cause more damage to the eye. Pour about a litre (1¾ pints) of warm water gently over the affected eye(s). Using a piece of cotton wool soaked in warm water, wipe around but not on the eye, removing any debris or discharge.

Treatment
Depending on the cause of the problem, the vet may prescribe antibiotics in the form of eye ointments or drops, and/or anti-inflammatory drugs, either topical (applied directly into the eye) or by mouth. Any such treatment must be given regularly, as directed, and the course should be completed or the problem may prove extremely difficult to clear up, and may recur regularly.

RELATED CONDITIONS WHICH MAY PRODUCE SIMILAR SYMPTOMS

Several other conditions can cause reddening of the eye, and it may also be the result of a foreign object in the cat's eye. It is therefore important that you have your cat examined by a vet before attempting any treatments.

Cataract

An opacity of the lens (or the capsule that surrounds it), that may affect one or both eyes, making it difficult for the cat to see things normally. Most cataracts get gradually worse.

Symptoms

A slight greying of the eyes is quite normal as a cat grows older, but it may also be the first indication that a cataract is developing. Where the cataracts are hereditary or caused by the dam's poor diet, they will start to appear when a kitten is just a few weeks old, and worsen progressively until the cat is totally blind. This is usually at two to three years of age, but may happen to cats as young as one.

DIAGNOSING CATARACTS

The cat's eyes will be examined using an ophthalmoscope. 👁

A poor diet during a dam's pregnancy can lead to the development of cataracts.

As the condition worsens, the affected cat will have greater difficulty leading a normal life. She may bump into objects, such as furniture and doors, and will be extremely anxious and stressed in unfamiliar surroundings.

Underlying causes

Many cats develop cataracts in their old age. Others have hereditary cataracts, while some cataracts develop due to poor nutrition of the dam in pregnancy. Diabetes mellitus (see p.24) is a common cause of cataracts in cats. Cataracts may be caused by a severe trauma, which disturbs the circulation within the eye, although this is extremely unlikely.

Owner action

Any cat suspected of suffering from cataracts must be examined by a vet as soon as possible.

Treatment

Depending on what the vet finds in the eye examination, the cat may be sent for further examination by a veterinary eye specialist, and surgery may be necessary to remove the affected lens(es).

HOMEOPATHIC TREATMENT:
Treat the cloudy lens – sulphur. In cases involving injury or an old cat – conium. Where the condition has degenerated following surgery – senega. For long-term treatment – silicea 30. Ask your vet for advice.

COST
If surgery is involved, the costs may be quite high.

Blindness

Inability to see clearly, or not able to see anything at all.

Symptoms
Your cat may bump into furniture and objects for no apparent reason. It is also quite common for an elderly cat to have more problems with her eyesight in bright light and also in darkness, and she may be reluctant to venture out at such times.

Underlying causes
A variety, from injury to hereditary diseases and conditions. As cats age, it is quite common for a bluish colour to appear in the eyes; this is a normal consequence of ageing, as the lens of the eye deteriorates, and may lead to deterioration of the cat's eyesight.

Treatment
Totally dependent upon the causes of the sight loss, but many cases of total blindness are not treatable.

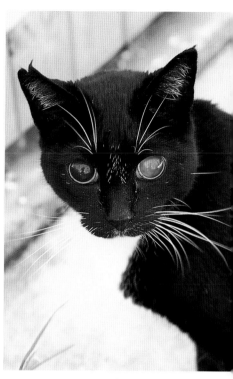

Cloudy or opaque eyes in a cat should be examined by a vet without delay.

DIAGNOSING BLINDNESS

The vet will use an ophthalmoscope to examination the cat's eyes. This has a built-in light with several filters and lenses which can be used to examine both the internal and external eye.

Corneal ulceration

URGENCY INDICATOR

Not life-
threatening, but
eye damage can
have serious
consequences, so
seek veterinary
advice.

An ulcer on the cornea, formed when the surface, which is usually very smooth, becomes damaged.

Symptoms
These include increased blinking, reddened eye, increased tear production, discomfort or pain, dislike of bright lights, a change of colour in the cornea (to an opaque blue-grey) and swollen conjunctiva (the membrane that covers the front of the eye).

DIAGNOSING CORNEAL ULCERATION

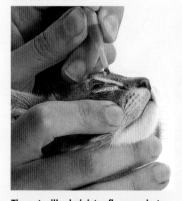

The vet will administer fluoroscein to the eye, which will stick to the ulcer, but run off the unaffected areas of the cornea. Ultraviolet light shone into the eye will make the dye fluoresce and enable the ulcer to be seen.

HOMEOPATHIC TREATMENT: Mercurial remedies, taken orally, may be effective. Ask your vet for advice.

Underlying causes
The damage to the cornea may be due to a scratch, a foreign body in the eye, an infection, a tumour, or damage caused by ingrowing eyelids. One type of ulcer is caused by *Pseudomonas* bacteria, and these ulcers are capable of spreading at such a fast rate, and are so aggressive, that they are known as 'melting ulcers'.

Any cat can suffer from corneal ulcers, particularly ageing cats. The ulcers are very painful and can soon spread, so must be treated by a vet as soon as possible. Some ulcers can rupture the cornea, causing extremely serious damage.

Owner action
It is best not to attempt any treatment of your cat's eyes; leave this to the vet, as you can easily cause serious and often irreparable damage.

Treatment
Any foreign body found in the eye will be removed by the vet, and antibiotics will be administered for infection. As the problem will cause the cat some discomfort, an Elizabethan collar may need to be fitted to prevent the eye being rubbed, which would cause further damage.

In a small minority of cases, where the corneal ulcer will not heal, the affliction may be treated surgically, either by cauterizing the ulcer or surgically removing damaged tissue around it. A flap of healthy conjunctiva may have to be fixed over the ulcer for a few days.

COST
Eye damage can need specialist veterinary treatment, and this could be expensive.

Feline chlamydial infection

Infection with *Chlamydia psittaci*, a bacterium, which causes conjunctivitis. Most common in young kittens (one to nine months of age).

Symptoms
Conjunctivitis (reddened eyes), and a thick ocular discharge. Sneezing and a nasal discharge are also often observed.

Underlying causes
Cats become infected by *Chlamydia psittaci* which is spread by other infected cats in their bodily discharges.

Owner action
Any eye infection must receive veterinary treatment urgently.

Treatment
Antibiotics will be prescribed. The whole course must be completed.

DIAGNOSING FELINE CHLAMYDIAL INFECTION
Laboratory analysis of blood and/or discharge.

COST
The costs of antibiotics are quite low.

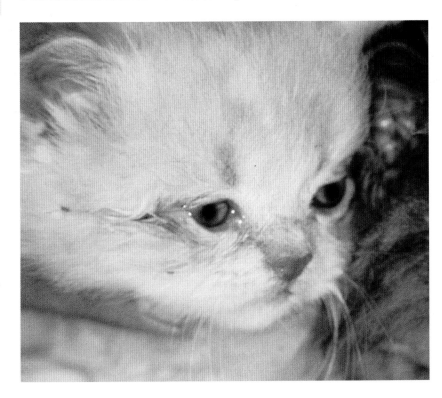

Feline chlamydial infection is common in kittens between one and nine months old. This 6-week-old Persian kitten shows signs of infection.

Abnormal tear production

HOMEOPATHIC TREATMENT:
Euphrasia, taken orally, is one of the most useful treatments for this condition. Your vet will advise you.

COST
A common condition, and if treated early it should not be expensive.

Overflowing of tears onto the cat's face, known as epiphora. Tears are one of nature's ways of flushing dirt and debris from the eyes, working together with the eyelids, and play an important role in keeping the eyes healthy.

Symptoms
Tears normally drain away through the tear duct, a tube-like vessel which connects the eye with the nose. When this flow is impeded, the tears overflow onto the cat's face. It is most obvious on cats with white faces. The condition is more common in the flat-faced breeds, such as the Persian cat, and cats with large, droopy eyelids also tend to suffer from epiphora more than the average cat.

Underlying causes
The usual cause of epiphora is one or both tear ducts being blocked. This blockage could be due to an infection, facial injury, a foreign body becoming lodged in the tear duct, scarring following an injury, or excessive mucus production. Some pedigree long-haired breeds are particularly prone to blockages of the tear ducts. Alternatively, the tear ducts may be unable to function correctly due to a congenital defect (one present from birth). Irritation of the eye may also cause abnormal tear production.

Owner action
Any cat with a persistently weepy eye or showing signs of tear-staining should be examined by a vet.

Treatment
Where the problem is caused by a lack of drainage, the vet may decide to anaesthetize or heavily sedate the cat, and wash out the blocked tear duct using a canula, a very fine tube attached to a syringe. Where the cause of the problem is an infection, antibiotics will be prescribed – ointment, drops or medicine by mouth.

A cat's eyes should be washed regularly with warm water to remove debris from the area before it can become a problem. This is particularly important if the cat is one of the breeds or types more susceptible to this condition. Prevention is better than cure.

If abnormal tear production is caused by infection, antibiotic cream and regular washing will help ease the condition.

DIAGNOSING ABNORMAL TEAR PRODUCTION

To observe the amount of drainage from an eye, the vet can put fluoroscein (a dye) into the affected eye(s). If the tear ducts are draining the eyes as they should be, the dye will then come down the cat's nostrils.

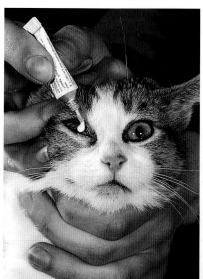

Glaucoma

A build-up of fluid in the eye leading to the tension of the fluid contents of the eye increasing.

Symptoms

Eventually swelling and bulging of the affected eye(s), and blindness. The cat will be in pain and may shy away from light, as the condition makes the pupils dilate excessively and continuously.

Underlying causes

Glaucoma is usually caused by a disease of the eye, the most common being lens dislocation. This is where the lens in the eye moves forward, possibly due to trauma.

Owner action

Never try to treat eye problems at home. Seek veterinary treatment.

Treatment

Depending on the underlying cause and severity of the condition, surgery may be needed to relieve the pressure and also to clear the blockage. In some cases, drug therapy is effective. The drugs used reduce tear production, dilate the pupil and help to improve the drainage from the eye.

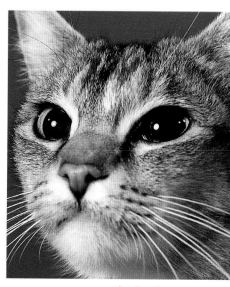

Dilated pupils are one of the sypmtoms of this condition. While not life-threatening glaucoma will cause your cat some discomfort.

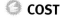 **HOMEOPATHIC TREATMENT:**
Symphytum and helleborus taken orally. Your vet will advise you on this.

⏱ COST

If surgery is involved, costs will be higher than for drug therapy.

DIAGNOSING GLAUCOMA

The vet will physically examine the cat's eyes. You may be referred to a veterinary eye specialist, and this vet may measure the pressure in the cat's eyes.

Ear conditions

The ear is made up of three parts.

● **The pinna (plural pinnae).** This is the outer part of the ear (the flap) which collects and funnels sounds to the ear drum, which changes these sounds to vibrations. The ear drum is a white sheet of tissue stretched across the ear canal.

● **The middle ear.** This part of the ear contains the ossicles (ear bones), and these transmit the vibrations from the ear drum to the inner ear.

● **The inner ear.** This is where the vibrations are translated into electrical signals, and these signals are then transmitted to the brain, which interprets them as sounds.

Any of these parts can, and sometimes do, cause problems in a cat. Some breeds of cat, particularly blue-eyed, white-coated breeds, are predisposed to hereditary ear problems. The gene responsible for this coloration often also causes deafness.

Canker (Otitis)

Inflammation of the skin lining the ear. Otitis is one of the most common conditions seen by vets in cats, and may occur in one or both ears.

Symptoms

May include regular ear-scratching and head-shaking, a discharge or smell from the ear, reddening of the inner ear flap and/or the ear hole. The cat may hiss at anyone who touches her around the ear.

Underlying causes

Normally, the amount of wax produced in a cat's ear is exactly the same amount that is lost naturally. Much of the wax is lost through evaporation of the water from the wax. Problems occur when the ears do not get proper ventilation and the wax builds up. This excess wax causes irritation, and the ear is stimulated to produce even more wax. This leads to ideal conditions for normally harmless fungi and bacteria to grow and prosper. Ear mites (see p.59), foreign bodies in the ear and skin problems can also cause otitis.

Owner action

Any cat showing any of the symptoms of irritated ears should by taken as soon as possible for examination by a vet: immediately if you suspect that your cat may have a foreign body lodged in her ear. *Never* attempt to remove any such blockage yourself, as you may damage the cat's ear permanently. Do not put any liquid, ointment or other medication inside the cat's ears without the express direction of your vet, and do not attempt to put any solid object inside the cat's ear, including cotton buds, which may also damage the ear. Even the discharge from the cat's ear should not be interfered with until your vet has had a chance to see it, as this may give the vet some clues about the ear problem.

Treatment

Treatment may include having the ear syringed (washed out), or the application of a topical medicine (one put directly into the ear), such as ear drops or ointment. More than one of these medicines will often be needed: one for, say, ear mites, and another (an anti-inflammatory) for the irritation that the mites are causing. Whatever medications are prescribed, it is important that you administer them exactly as you are instructed, and finish the course of treatment. In serious cases of recurring otitis, the vet may have to operate on your cat to improve the ear ventilation.

URGENCY INDICATOR

Even though otitis is not a serious condition, if it is not properly treated it can become chronic, causing severe problems, and possibly damage to parts of the ear and to the cat's hearing.

HOMEOPATHIC TREATMENT: Psorinum, sulphur or conium given internally will make the ear hostile to mites. Ask the vet for advice.

COST

Unlikely to be high if caught in the early stages.

DIAGNOSING CANKER

The vet uses an instrument called an otoscope to see inside the cat's ear. The otoscope is fitted with cone-shaped ends of differing sizes, enabling the device to fit snugly into the cat's ear canal. It has a magnifying lens and its own light source. The vet can use it to examine the lining of the ear canal, and the ear drum.

When a cat is suffering from cancer, it may not be possible for your vet to use an otoscope properly because of the build-up of wax. If ear mites have caused the irritation, these may not be seen by the otoscope, as they dislike light, and hide under bits of wax when the light is shone in the ear.

Your vet may take a sample of the discharge and/or wax from the ear, and send these for laboratory examination. This will help pinpoint both the problem and the correct and most efficient treatment.

Aural haematoma

URGENCY INDICATOR

Aural haematoma is painful for the affected cat, and curing it can be quite complicated, so treatment should be started as soon as possible. The condition worsens over time, as the haematoma increases in size and becomes more difficult to treat.

HOMEOPATHIC TREATMENT:
Arnica or hamamelis given orally. Your vet will advise you on homeopathic treatments.

COST
This condition can be difficult to treat, and many different treatments may have to be tried before the condition clears up completely, so costs may be quite high.

A blood blister on the ear flap.

Symptoms
A lump under the skin of the pinna, which may or may not be painful to the cat.

Underlying causes
When a cat scratches her ears and shakes her head in response to irritation, perhaps caused by fleas or mites, or an ear infection, she may scratch too hard, shake it too vigorously or bang the ear flap against a solid object, causing a blood blister. This is the accumulation of fluid between the layers of skin in the ear flap, around the cartilage sheet. In some cases aural haematoma may be caused by the cat's immune system reacting to an infection.

Owner action
Although aural haematoma is not life-threatening, you should consult the vet as soon as possible, as any delay can make the condition worse.

Treatment
It may take the vet more than one attempt to cure the aural haematoma, and different treatments may be tried. These may include drawing the fluid out with a syringe (aspiration), inserting a drainage tube into the haematoma and leaving it in place for several weeks; or even operating on the cat, using a general anaesthetic, and cutting open the ear to flush out the contents of the haematoma.

Antibiotics and/or painkillers are also usually prescribed, and the cat may have to wear an Elizabethan collar.

DIAGNOSING AURAL HAEMATOMA

The vet will examine the cat's ear externally, and internally using an otoscope. The vet is also likely to examine the rest of the cat, to discover what has made her scratch herself so vigorously. The irritants may be fleas or other parasites, or perhaps an ear infection.

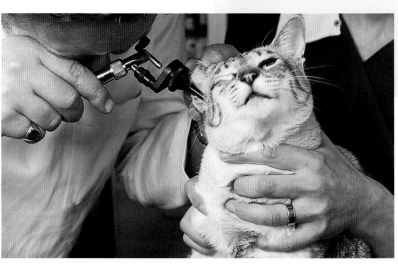

Ear mites

Insect parasites common in cats.

Symptoms
Persistent ear-scratching.

Underlying causes
Ear mites, *Otodectes cynotis*, which are common in cats and also in wild rodents.

Owner action
Seek veterinary advice in all cases of ear mites, loss of balance etc. All animals that have been in contact with the infected cat must also be treated, as ear mites can infect other animals who may not show any symptoms for some time.

Treatment
In mild cases, ear drops will be prescribed. Anti-inflammatory drugs may also be prescribed if the cat's ears are irritated due to the action of the mites.

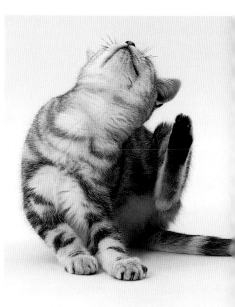

A cat suffering from ear mites will spend considerable time scratching her ears.

URGENCY INDICATOR

If left untreated, the irritation caused by mites will cause the cat to scratch, sometimes until her ears actually bleed. The mites can move down the ear canal and infect the middle ear; such an infection will cause the affected animal to lose her sense of balance. The cat may be unable to hold her head straight or, in more serious cases, may constantly fall over.

HOMEOPATHIC TREATMENT: Psorinum or sulphur will help relieve irritation, but normal veterinary treatments must be used to get rid of the mites.

DIAGNOSING EAR MITES

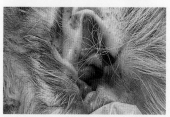

A build-up of wax in the ears, dotted with black specks, is an indication that a cat may have ear mites; the black specks are probably spots of dried blood. The ear mites are usually white or colourless and are not visible to the naked eye – a magnifying lens or otoscope is required, although otoscopes may not be able to detect them as the mites hide under pieces of wax.

COST
Mites are easily treated if caught early enough, and so the cost will be quite low.

RELATED CONDITIONS WHICH MAY PRODUCE SIMILAR SYMPTOMS

Many similar conditions can give the general symptoms of an ear-mite infestation, so it is essential that your vet diagnoses the problem and treats it accordingly.

Deafness

Partial or complete loss of hearing.

Symptoms
The cat may fail to respond to verbal stimuli, or appear to sleep very soundly, not waking when you call her.

Underlying causes
There are many different causes of deafness in a cat. Deafness is not itself a disease, but a symptom of a problem or disease.

The problem could occur anywhere along the route taken by sounds before they arrive at the brain. This could include a physical blockage of the ear canal, by either a physical agent, swelling(s) or even small tumours, known as polyps. The ear drum itself may be damaged, as may the ossicles. There may be a build-up of fluid in the middle ear, or the problem may be associated with old age. Some animals are born with deformities and abnormalities of the ear. In some breeds, especially those with white fur and blue eyes, deafness is a known and almost expected problem as the gene responsible for this coloration often also causes deafness, but deafness can occur in any breed.

Owner action
It can often be surprisingly difficult to notice that your cat actually has a hearing problem, since many compensate for their hearing loss, for example by looking more intently at their owners. If you suspect that there may be a problem, try speaking to your cat when she has her back turned, or when her attention is on something she has seen. Also try different types, volumes and pitches of sound.

If you feel that your cat fails these tests, or that they are inconclusive, seek veterinary help.

Treatment
If there is a blockage, the vet will remove this, and, if possible, treat any underlying problems that may originally have caused the blockage.

If your cat is profoundly and permanently deaf, you will have to face the dilemma that keeping a deaf cat produces. Many people feel that it is possible for a deaf cat to live a fairly normal life. Your vet will be able to offer advice and guidance on individual cases.

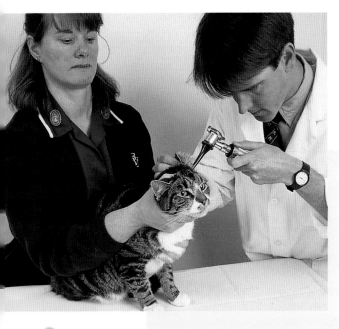

🔵 COST
This will depend on the cause of the deafness, as well as the number of tests needed to diagnose the underlying problem.

DIAGNOSING DEAFNESS

Your vet will examine the cat's ears for obvious physical problems and, if these are not found, he will carry out more tests, sometimes including electronic hearing tests.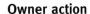

Ear flap wounds

Scratches or tears to the ear flaps.

Symptoms
Any ear wound, no matter how minor, is likely to bleed a great deal. Even if the actual wound does not cause the cat any real pain, the irritation of blood running down the ear is likely to cause her to scratch at her ear and shake her head.

Underlying causes
Ear flaps are often bitten and scratched when cats fight, and some cats, particularly farm cats, may injure their ear flaps in their usual day-to-day life.

Owner action
With someone restraining the cat, the wounds should be cleaned, using saline solution made by dissolving one table-spoon of table salt in 0.5 litre (18 fl oz) of warm water. Once cleaned, it will be possible to see the extent of the damage to the ear flap. If this is significant, then veterinary treatment should be sought, as the wounds may need suturing (stitching).

Treatment
After cleaning with saline solution, minor wounds should be covered with antiseptic ointment, cream or powder. If the wounds look inflamed within a few days of the injury, consult the vet, as the cat may need treatment with antibiotics.

To keep the dressing on the ear flap in place, it may be necessary to cut one leg from a pair of tights and, once some padding has been placed around the affected ear flap, place the leg of the tights over the cat's head, in such a way that the ear is held flat to the cat's head. While this works in some cats, others will quickly scratch at it to remove it, in which case you should seek advice from the vet.

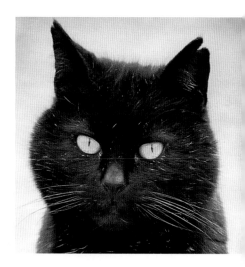

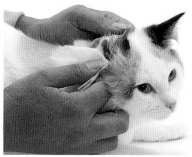

HOMEOPATHIC TREATMENT:
Symphytum and helleborus taken orally. Your vet will advise you on this.

COST
Minor ear injuries, treated adequately soon after the injury occurs, will cost little to treat.

Top: **Ear flap wounds are not usually serious but need to be treated with a saline solution before they become infected.**

Bottom: **Apply ear drops to the inside of the ear, and then massage the ear gently to allow the drops to do their work.**

The skin

The cat's body is covered by a protective layer of skin. It is composed of three layers:

● **the epidermis, the outermost layer;**
● **the dermis, the middle layer; and**
● **the hypodermis, the innermost layer.**

Skin serves a number of functions. It keeps out foreign bodies and keeps in moisture. It also helps to regulate the cat's body temperature. It manufactures vitamin D, and contains receptors for pain, temperature and pressure. The hair and pigment in the skin protect the body from the harmful effects of ultraviolet radiation, and the skin also contains sebaceous and sweat glands. Cats do sweat, but they do not use sweat to help control their body temperature as humans do.

Claws, pads and hair are special modifications of the skin. Hair is formed from epidermis, and grows through a tube known as the hair follicle. Each hair follicle has a sebaceous gland to lubricate and waterproof the hair and the skin. These glands produce a scent that the cat uses as a marker for its territory. The sebaceous glands also produce hormones called pheromones that help attract cats of the opposite sex.

There are three types of hair:

● **Guard hairs** The long hairs of the top coat of the cat's fur, which provide the waterproofing of the cat's coat.
● **Undercoat or wool hairs** These are shorter than the guard hairs, and trap air to keep the cat warm. They make up most of the coat of a kitten, and there are more wool hairs on an adult cat in winter than in summer.
● **Vibrissae** Hairs that are sensitive to touch, the 'whiskers' around the mouth and eyes, and on each cheek.

WARNING: NEVER CUT THE VIBRISSAE WITHOUT GOOD REASON.

Moulting is when the cat sheds her hair each season to have a coat suitable for that time of year: a thick winter coat and a thinner summer one. Sometimes larger than normal amounts of hair are lost; this is known as seasonal abnormality moulting and is quite common. It often leads to sections of the cat's body, usually her flanks, being almost totally without hair, and the hair usually grows back at the time of the next moult.

WARNING: MANY OF THE SKIN CONDITIONS WHICH MAY AFFECT YOUR CAT ARE ZOONOTIC, AND SO COULD ALSO AFFECT YOU.

Alopecia

Abnormal hair loss.

**URGENCY
INDICATOR**

Although
unsightly (to us)
and annoying to
the affected cat,
this is not a life-
threatening
condition.

**HOMEOPATHIC
TREATMENT:**
Alumen, selenium,
thallium and ustilago
can all be useful for
treating alopecia.
Ask your vet for
advice.

COST
Unlikely to be high,
although some skin
conditions that cause
alopecia such as
hypersensitivity,
which will require
quite extensive
treatment until the
cause is found, can
be quite difficult to
cure and require
long-term treatment.

Symptoms
*Affected areas will have little or no fur
covering, and the skin may be blotchy,
broken and sore. Sometimes, quite large
areas of the cat's body may be affected.
Where the hair on the abdomen becomes
extremely thin, or disappears
completely, this is known as feline
symmetric alopecia.*

Underlying causes
It is thought that stress can cause hair loss
in cats, as well as in humans. In cats, this is

DIAGNOSING ALOPECIA

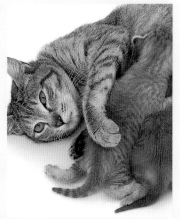

**Alopecia is most evident when a queen
is raising a litter of kittens. For
accurate diagnosis of skin complaints,
the vet will need to take 'skin scrapes'
for laboratory analysis. This will
involve scraping a small piece of
skin from the affected area of the cat,
which will be examined under a
microscope for parasites, fungi
or other organisms.**

most evident when the queen is pregnant
or raising a litter of kittens, and therefore
lactating, when she is likely to lose much of
her hair. The hair almost always re-grows to
its normal condition.

When fleas bite a cat to feed on her
blood, they secrete saliva to prevent the
blood from clotting, and some cats develop
an allergy to this saliva. This affliction is
referred to as 'flea allergic dermatitis', and
will cause the cat to scratch herself even
more than she would do for a normal flea
infestation. This leads to hair loss, often
over quite a large part of the cat's body, in
particular the flanks, tail and the rump. This
condition may also lead to another skin
condition – folliculitis, caused by a bacterium, and this may further intensify the
problem. See p.65–73 for information on
fleas and other parasites.

Owner action
As some skin complaints may be zoonotic
(that is, may cross to humans), care should
be taken that you do not catch them.
Commonsense hygiene precautions and
practices should be followed; never handle
the affected cat without washing your
hands with a top quality soap, and never
allow children to handle any such affected
cat in any way.

Treatment
This depends entirely upon the underlying
cause. If the problem is a parasite infestation, the vet will prescribe powders, ointments or creams. In some cases, it may be
possible to treat such infestations by inject-
ing the cat with one of the new drugs on
the market.

Food allergies

Cats may develop an allergy to one or more of the contents of their feed. Itchy skin will be a symptom.

Symptoms
If your cat spends considerable time scratching at her coat, then you should seek veterinary advice.

Underlying causes
Food allergies are caused by one or more of the contents of the feed, and there is much debate and controversy surrounding the subject. Cow's milk, wheat and even some meats have been known to cause allergies in cats and other domestic animals.

Owner action
Always feed a top quality diet, and only change it if necessary. Changing the diet should be done gradually over a period of seven to ten days.

Treatment
In some cases, the cat will be put on a strict diet, with different food constituents being fed at different times, in order to find out which constituent(s) cause the problem. In other cases, drug therapy may be called for.

The best way to avoid food allergies is to provide your cat with a top quality diet.

DIAGNOSING ALLERGIES

In many cases, the vet will need to take a blood or skin sample from the affected cat. The taking of a skin sample is an uncomfortable, though not painful, experience for the cat, in which the vet will use a scalpel to scrape a small amount of the surface layer of skin off the cat's body. This sample will then be sent for laboratory analysis, in order to identify the cause of the cat's condition. The laboratory procedures will include microscopic examination, in order to eliminate or confirm the possibility of mites or a fungal infection, such as ringworm (see p.70).

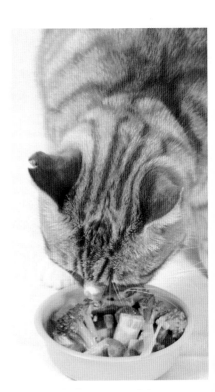

RELATED CONDITIONS WHICH MAY PRODUCE SIMILAR SYMPTOMS

Alopecia (see p.63).

Fleas

Fleas are insects that live as parasites on other animals. Even the most pampered cats can suffer from the unwanted attentions of parasites, either internal (endoparasites) or external (ectoparasites).

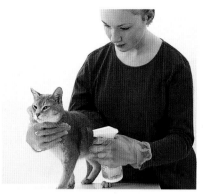

When using flea sprays, it is important that you wear rubber gloves to protect yourself.

Symptoms

Fleas are the most common ectoparasite; they bite their host and then feed on the blood that appears at the bite site. This area will show an inflammatory reaction, and will cause a certain amount of irritation to the cat.

DIAGNOSING PARASITE INFESTATION

The vet will examine the fleas on your cat under a microscope. Identification of the flea can be carried out by the appearance of the flea's head, where the presence or otherwise of 'combs' is used to identify the particular species.

Underlying causes

By far the most common flea to infect cats is the so-called 'cat flea' (*Ctenocephalides felis*), although they may be infected with the dog flea (*Ctenocephalides canis*). Cats are also liable to infestations of the rabbit flea (*Spilopsyllus cuniculi*) and the hedgehog flea (*Archaeopsylla erinacei*). Rabbit fleas group together around the ear, and hedgehog fleas are very large in comparison to the other types of fleas that your cat may catch.

Owner action

In all cases of flea infestation, all the cat's bedding must be removed and treated, and the household carpets treated, along with other household pets, in order to break the life cycle of the flea. Treating only the affected cat(s) is not treating the whole problem. Treatment of the household will prevent flea eggs hatching, and the larvae developing.

Use anti-flea preparations to treat all bedding and the cat's bed itself. Do *not* use such powders and sprays where a queen is still feeding her kittens, as there is a danger of poisoning the litter.

Treatment

There are many insecticidal preparations available from the vet, in the form of sprays, powders, impregnated collars or shampoos. The vet may suggest a natural remedy, such as a herbal preparation, or a collar impregnated with such a preparation. In the USA, diatomaceous earth (the fossilized remains of a single-celled alga) is popular as a flea treatment. It is dusted on affected cats and also on carpets, rugs, furniture, pet beds and bedding, and anywhere that fleas and/or their eggs may collect. This material is entirely safe for humans and pets, but is deadly to fleas and many other insects, even in their larval stage. The fine particles in the diatomaceous earth attack the wax coating that covers the exoskeleton of the fleas, and the affected fleas dry out and die.

URGENCY INDICATOR

Not life-threatening, though very annoying to all concerned.

HOMEOPATHIC TREATMENT:

Sulphur can be given weekly to help prevent flea infestations, while pulex will soothe the irritation caused by the fleas. Ask your vet for advice.

COST

Flea treatments are quite effective and relatively cheap.

Mites

Mites are insect ectoparasites. There are several types commonly found on cats, and they all have unpleasant effects. See also ear mites, p.59. The mite *Sarcoptes scabiei* causes sarcoptic mange in cats, leading to alopecia (see p.63) and pruritis (intense itching), especially on elbows, hocks and ear flaps.

Symptoms
The first sign of mange is persistent scratching, even though there is no obvious cause such as fleas. Eventually, the skin becomes very red and sore, a symptom that is easier to see in cats with a white coat. As the disease progresses, these sores cause baldness and the sores themselves become worse.

Underlying causes
Sarcoptes scabiei is invisible to the naked eye. Cats can become infected with this mite by direct contact with other infected animals, such as rodents, or simply by being on infected ground. This type of mange is very common in cats.

Owner action
Be warned – mange can be contracted by humans (in humans, the condition is known as scabies). Take commonsense precautions to ensure that neither you nor your family will contract scabies, washing your hands after handling any cat believed to be infected with mites, or, even better, using disposable latex gloves.

Treatment
A wash that kills parasites must be applied to the affected areas. Use the wash under veterinary advice only. The cat's living quarters must be thoroughly treated by soaking in a strong solution of disinfectant or bleach, which must be washed off before

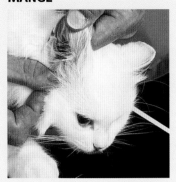
any cat is returned to the area. Veterinary drug companies are continually producing new topical applications to combat this problem; your vet will be able to advise you on the availability and effectiveness of these products.

'Walking dandruff'

The mite *Cheyletiella* causes the cat's skin to become dry and flaky.

Symptoms

The cat's skin appears dry and flaky, just like dandruff in humans; the 'dandruff' is particularly pronounced along the back and flanks of the cat who may, or may not, scratch at the affected areas.

Underlying causes

Cheyletiella is invisible to the naked eye. It is caught from contact with an infected cat.

Owner action

Ensure that other family pets (such as dogs and rabbits) are treated at the same time as your cat, as this mite will infect them too. Look after yourself and your family by using commonsense hygiene precautions, such as washing hands after handling the affected animal, and not allowing children to handle such cats at all.

Treatment

A wash that kills the parasites will need to be applied regularly over a period of four to five weeks.

URGENCY INDICATOR

Modern anti-parasite drugs are effective and relatively cheap.

HOMEOPATHIC TREATMENT:
Symphytum and helleborus taken orally. Your vet will advise you on this.

COST

Minor ear injuries, treated adequately soon after the injury occurs, will cost little to treat.

DIAGNOSING 'WALKING DANDRUFF'

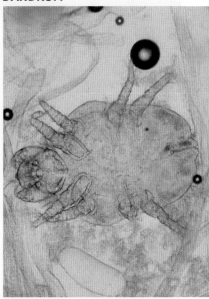

The vet will examine samples of the affected skin under a microscope.

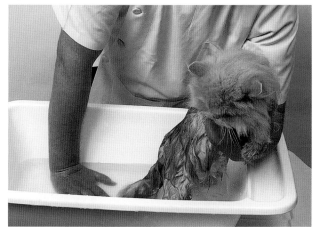

RELATED CONDITIONS WHICH MAY PRODUCE SIMILAR SYMPTOMS

Ringworm (see p.70) may produce similar symptoms.

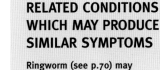

With many skin problems, it will be necessary to bath your cat using a prescribed shampoo.

Ticks

Ticks are insect ectoparasites. By far the most common types of tick to affect cats in the United Kingdom are the sheep tick (*Ixodes ricinus*), and the hedgehog tick (*Ixodes hexagonus*).

Symptoms

The cat will spend more time scratching herself, and you will be able to see the ticks, which look like swollen grains of brown rice.

Underlying causes

Ticks are ectoparasites that most cats will catch at some stage. They are carriers of certain bacteria, harmful to many animals, and they also carry a range of diseases, such as Lyme's disease, which can affect humans. Ticks may be contracted from other cats, or other animal species including dogs and rabbits, or even from vegetation which can be infested with them.

Owner action

When an infestation of ticks has been discovered on your cat, all her bedding must be removed, and preferably burned, and her bed thoroughly disinfected. Use tick powder or spray, available from the vet, to treat all bedding and the bed. Do *not* use such powders and sprays where a queen is still feeding her kittens, unless the vet gives absolute assurances that it is suitable for use in this situation. With most of these powders, there is a danger of poisoning the litter.

Treatment

Ticks are rather more difficult to deal with than fleas, but they do respond to some sprays and powders. In some countries, these may only be available from vets as they are classed as 'prescription only medicines', whereas in other countries they are freely available at pharmacies and even

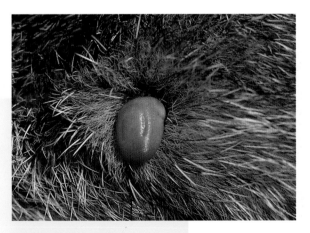

DIAGNOSING TICK INFESTATION

Physical examination of the cat's coat will reveal the ticks, which may then be identified.

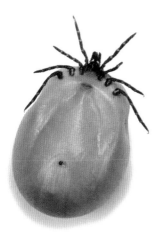

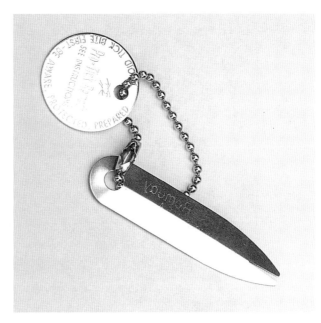

Ticks are eight-legged creatures, related to spiders and are at their most visible when engorged with cat's blood.

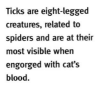

pet shops. The use of organophosphates, compounds found in flea and tick powders, on domestic animals such as cats is banned in many countries.

Ticks attach themselves to their host by burying their head under the top layers of the host's skin, and use their mouthparts to feed from the host. Care must be taken when removing ticks to ensure that the mouthparts are completely removed from the cat's skin, otherwise infection and abscesses can occur; never simply pull ticks out. Paint alcohol on the tick using a fine paint brush, and the tick should have died and dropped off within 24 hours; if not, repeat the process.

Although some authorities suggest that ticks can be burned off with a lighted cigarette, this should never be attempted. It is all too easy to burn the cat with the cigarette and the alcohol method is much

more effective, with none of the dangers.

A number of devices are now on the market that have been specifically designed to remove ticks, due mainly to concern about the spread of Lyme's disease in humans. Among these is a type of sprung forceps that grip the tick around the head; the device is then gently twisted backwards and forwards until the tick comes out. I have tested several such implements, and have had 100 per cent success with each; I now always keep one in my first aid kit.

RELATED CONDITIONS WHICH MAY PRODUCE SIMILAR SYMPTOMS

Owners may mistake warts and other growths for ticks, or vice versa.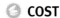

A number of devices have been designed for the effective removal of ticks. Always keep one in your first aid kit.

🔵 **COST**

Modern treatments for tick infestations are highly effective, while their cost is quite low.

Ringworm

A fungal infection of the cat's epidermis and the hair fibres in the skin, and not, as some people believe, an actual worm.

The condition is highly infectious, so veterinary treatment should be sought in all cases.

Symptoms
The affected cat may spend time scratching herself, or rubbing against solid objects. There will be round areas of hair loss.

Underlying causes
The most common fungi responsible for ringworm in cats are *Microsporum canis*, *Microsporum gypseum* and *Trichophyton mentagrophytes*. The spores of these fungi may be wind-borne or found in the soil. All are highly infectious.

Owner action
Some of the fungi that can cause ringworm in cats are zoonotic. Care must be taken to ensure that neither you nor your family become infected.

Treatment
Ringworm is usually treated by washing the animal in a fungicidal wash prescribed by the vet, such as enilconazole. In some cases, the vet may 'paint' the affected areas with tincture of iodine, or apply an ointment (Whitfield's ointment) consisting of salicylic and benzoic acid, which kills the fungus and prevents its spores escaping into the environment. All topical treatments (those applied directly onto the affected area) must be repeated for a full cure.

DIAGNOSING RINGWORM

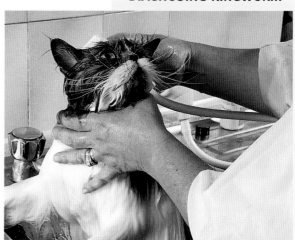

Ringworm appears as small round areas of hair loss. It is usually possible to see the fungus around the edges of the affected area, often as whitish, scaly skin. It is usually treated with a fungicidal wash.

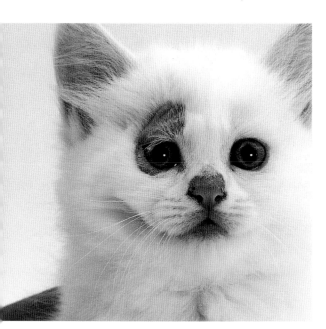

A Lilac Tonkinese kitten with ringworm infection on its head and face.

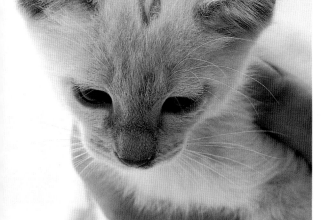

This kitten has lesions on its head caused by ringworm. The spores responsible for this condition are highly infectious to cats and can be carried on the wind or found in the soil.

HOMEOPATHIC TREATMENT: Depends upon the actual organism responsible for the condition. Bacillinium, berberis, chrysarobinum, sepia or tellurium may be effective. Ask the vet for advice.

COST

The ointments and other medicines used to cure ringworm are not expensive.

RELATED CONDITIONS WHICH MAY PRODUCE SIMILAR SYMPTOMS

Flea allergies (see p.65) and alopecia (see p.63).

Feline pyoderma

Bacterial infection of a cat's skin.

Symptoms
Vary depending on the underlying cause: see below.

DIAGNOSING FELINE PYODERMA

The vet will take skin scrapes to establish which bacterium is causing the pyoderma.

Regular grooming will help to prevent your cat developing this bacterial infection.

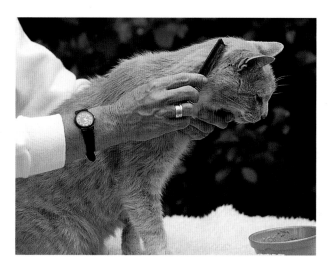

COST
The costs should be relatively low, but treatment may take some time so the costs will reflect this.

Underlying causes
A cat normally has a certain amount of 'friendly' bacteria on its skin which fight off infection. Occasionally, the friendly bacteria multiply to the extent that they begin to harm the cat. A bacterial infection of the cat's skin is known as pyoderma. This is a fairly rare condition in cats, but can cause a number of diseases including:

● **Acute moist dermatitis** Often referred to as 'wet eczema', this gives symptoms of inflamed, wet and painful sores. It is particularly common in long-haired cats, and is probably the result of other conditions, such as parasite infestations.

● **Callus pyoderma** The infection of the thick skin over the cat's bony protuberances, such as her elbows.

● **Inter-digital pyoderma** As the name suggests, this condition affects the skin between the cat's toes or digits, and is often triggered by the presence of a foreign body, such as a piece of salt grit or grass seed. Matted fur between the toes may also trigger this condition, as may irritant chemicals (very often the disinfectant or detergent used to clean the cat's bed).

Owner action
Ensure your cat is groomed on a regular basis; this will reveal pyoderma before it becomes severe.

Treatment
Antibiotics are used to treat all types of pyoderma. They may be in the form of shampoos, topical ointments or creams, or antibiotic medicines. The whole course of any antibiotics should be completed.

Seborrhoea

An abnormal/excessive secretion from the cat's sebaceous glands. Under normal circumstances, the skin renews cells at the same rate that cells die. When this balance becomes affected, as with this condition, new cells are not produced at the same rate as the old cells die off and the thickness of the skin is affected.

Symptoms
Areas of dead skin will become visible. These areas will appear flaky or greasy and may exhibit signs of inflammation.

DIAGNOSING SEBORRHOEA

Skin scrapes, blood tests and laboratory analysis of skin and hair samples will help the vet to diagnose and treat the problem.

Underlying causes
The causes may include pyoderma (see p.84), ectoparasite infestations, hot, dry conditions, use of incorrect shampoos and/or grooming techniques, nutritional disorders, hypothyroidism, Cushing's disease (see p.100), or maybe diabetes mellitus (see p.24).

Owner action
Regular grooming, a good diet and control of the cat's environment (avoiding dry, hot surroundings) will all help prevent this condition.

Treatment
Depending on the cause of the problem, treatment for seborrhoea may include antibiotics, especially if the condition has led to the cat developing pyoderma (see p.84), and anti-inflammatory drug therapy in cases where the cat's skin is extremely inflamed and sore. Often, simply adding fat (vegetable or animal) to a cat's diet will help a mild case of seborrhoea. If the condition is caused by a flea infestation, a course of anti-parasite powders, sprays or 'spot-ons' (drugs that are literally spotted on to the affected area) will be needed.

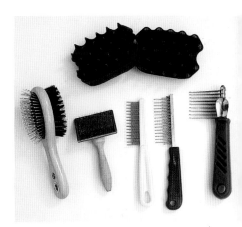

There are many different grooming tools available. Take care to choose those best suited to your needs.

Male cat problems

There are certain conditions and problems that only or mainly affect male cats, in particular their reproductive system.

The normal male cat has two testes or testicles in which spermatozoa are produced; these are contained in the scrotum, a pouch of skin. Spermatozoa are passed down to the epididymis, where they are stored. When the cat is mating, the spermatozoa pass through tubes to the urethra (the tube that carries urine away from the bladder), where they are mixed with fluid from the prostate and other glands. The mixture formed is known as semen, and is ejaculated through the cat's penis during mating.

Testosterone, the male sex hormone, is also produced by the testes, and it is this hormone which produces the secondary male characteristics, such as the tom's size, shape and voice.

Normally, a tom's testes descend into his scrotum at about ten days old, and the cat will reach sexual activity at between six and 12 months. Male cats are sexually active throughout the year, with only a minor seasonal change. Although a cat may be sexually mature at six months old, it is inadvisable to use him for stud (breeding) purposes until he is about 15 months old, and you have had the opportunity to evaluate his qualities fully. In breeds where there are some hereditary conditions or diseases, you should ensure that your cat has been examined by a vet and cleared of all such hereditary problems.

Although the age at which male cats cease to be fertile varies from breed to breed, seminal fluid quality will reduce from about seven years of age.

Sexual behaviour

Some toms will seek to mate even when a queen is not present.

Symptoms

The tom will be constantly restless, wanting to be let out. He may then not be seen for several days and nights. If confined to the human home, he will spend a lot of time scratching at doors and calling, often becoming extremely agitated. The tom may mount other animals, small children, and even the legs of human adults. From about six months of age, tom cats will start 'spraying', that is marking their territory (including furniture) with urine. This urine has an extremely powerful and unpleasant smell which is very difficult to clear from the human home. Consequently, most owners of tom cats choose to have them castrated.

Underlying causes

Such behaviour is linked to the androgens, the male sex hormones.

Owner action

There is very little that the owner can do in this situation.

Treatment

Neutering a tom will usually prevent him from spraying his urine to mark his territory, and will also stop him from wandering in search of queens. However, it is not unknown for a neutered tom to continue spraying. A castrated cat is less likely to get into fights with other toms, as most of these fights are over territory. Neutering may change the cat's nature, usually making him more home-loving.

If a cat's owner does not wish to have the cat castrated, or in cases where the cat will be used for breeding purposes at some time in its life, chemical control of the tom's sexual urges is possible. This is brought about by the administration, by a vet, of hormones that will suppress the normal release of testosterone (a male sex hormone). The most common drugs used are known as progestogens, which act like female hormones and reduce the tom's libido (sex drive) without affecting his fertility. These drugs may be given as a 'depot injection', where the effects of the injected drug last for some time, or as tablets on a daily basis.

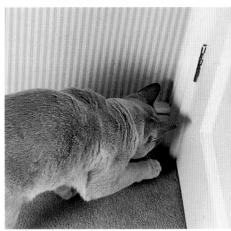

A tom cat which is constantly restless and wanting to go out could be demonstrating a high sex drive.

Aggression

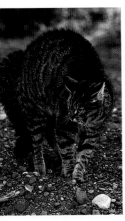

Cats which suddenly become aggressive for no apparent reason may benefit from being neutered.

There are many different types of aggression, each of which will require different treatment.

Symptoms
Your cat may suddenly change his attitude towards you, other members of your family or other animals. This may manifest itself in your cat attacking these people or animals.

Underlying causes
The different types of aggression are as follows:
- competitive
- dominance
- fear-induced
- maternal
- pain-induced
- pathophysiological
- play
- possessive
- predatory
- territorial

These types of aggression, with the exception of pathophysiological aggression, are behavioural in nature. Pathophysiological aggression is due to medical disorders.

Owner action
Try not to overreact to your cat's aggression, and seek veterinary advice on the problem. Remember never to leave small children around any aggressive animal.

Treatment
Neutering a tom will usually solve many of the aggressive behavioural problems he may be displaying.

Where a cat is castrated before reaching puberty, he may fail to develop his secondary sexual characteristics. It is also possible that such action will result in a change to the cat's metabolic rate, causing him to experience problems with his weight. However, where a cat is castrated after he has reached puberty, provided that proper dietary controls are exercised, there should be no major problems associated with the neutering.

Urolithiasis

A cat may develop stones in his urinary system (usually but not always in the bladder). These stones are known as uroliths, and the condition as urolithiasis. In severe cases the male cat's urine flow may be completely blocked, which could lead to acute renal (kidney) failure (see p.38).

Symptoms
Very little urine is passed by an affected cat, and what is passed is likely to be

Prostate problems

bloodstained. The cat will show severe discomfort and straining when urinating. In severe cases, the affected cat cannot pass any urine at all.

Underlying causes
The male cat's urethra is very narrow, and crystals form from the urine and block the urethra. This is known as a sabulous plug. This occurs as a result of the cat's diet.

Owner action
Your vet may prescribe a special diet for the cat, to prevent the condition recurring.

Treatment
The cat will be given a general anaesthetic, then a catheter is passed into his penis and the urethra is flushed out with Walpole's solution. In severe cases, the tom's penis to be amputated. Surgery may also be used to establish another opening through which the urine can be expelled. Where a cat suffers a secondary urinary infection as a result of urolithiasis, antibiotics may be used to treat this infection.

RELATED CONDITIONS WHICH MAY PRODUCE SIMILAR SIGNS
Bladder infections, for example cystitis (see p.36).

 HOMEOPATHIC TREATMENT:
Sarsaparilla and thlaspi bursa will both help to prevent the formation of uroliths. Ask your vet for advice.

🌟 COST
Any operation involving a general anaesthetic is likely to be quite costly.

The prostate gland is at the base of the male cat's bladder, where the urethra (the tube that carries urine away from the bladder) begins. The prostate gland produces secretions that combine with spermatozoa and secretions from other glands to form semen. Problems with the prostate gland can cause the cat to have great trouble urinating and even defecating.

Symptoms
May include incontinence, constipation, blood in the urine, a bleeding penis, pus from the penis, straining to pass feces and/or the production of ribbon-like feces.

DIAGNOSING PROSTATE PROBLEMS
The vet will carry out a physical examination of the cat's abdomen. Blood and/or pus samples may need to be obtained and analyzed. The vet may also carry out X-rays and ultrasound examinations.

Underlying causes
Sometimes, when a male cat is between six and ten years of age, the prostate begins to enlarge. This condition is known as hyperplasia, and is considered normal by many vets. Another cause is when harmful bacteria get into the prostate gland, and cause an infection; this is known as prostatitis.

Treatment
If the problem is hyperplasia, drug and/or hormone treatment may be given. In severe cases the vet may recommend that the affected cat is castrated. In cases of prostatitis, long-term courses of antibiotics may be used.

URGENCY INDICATOR

Because of the symptoms which this condition can cause, treatment is best started as soon as the problem is diagnosed.

 HOMEOPATHIC TREATMENT:
Agnus castus, conium and selenium may be effective for this condition. The vet will advise you.

🌟 COST
Depends on the severity of the problem, but costs are usually moderate.

Anal adenoma

Anorchia and cryptorchidism

Tumours around the anus, just under the skin. The adenoma is benign, that is, not malignant (fatal if left untreated), and there is a good chance of complete recovery. This condition is rare in cats, but not unknown.

Symptoms
The tumours feel 'knobbly' to the touch.

DIAGNOSING ANAL ADENOMAS

Physical examination, sometimes coupled with radiography.

Underlying causes
Anal adenomas are directly linked to the androgens (male sex hormones) present in older cats.

Owner action
There is nothing that the owner can do to help this condition.

Treatment
Anal adenomas can become very large and ulcerate, and the vet may decide to operate to improve the condition. As the tumour's growth depends upon the level of testosterone (a male sex hormone) in the cat's body, the vet may recommend treatment with hormones that will suppress the normal release of testosterone. The most common drugs used are known as progestogens, which act like female hormones, 'neutralizing' the level of testosterone in the cat. In some cases, the tom may have to be surgically castrated, and this will prevent the condition from recurring.

Where a cat's testes are both absent as a result of a natural phenomenon, the condition is known as anorchia. This is very rare. Cryptorchidism is when the testicles have not descended.

Symptoms
In normal male cats, both testes can be seen when the cat is a few weeks old. If this is not the case, then there could be a potentially serious problem, particularly if you intend to breed from or show the cat. Monorchids have one testicle that has descended, with the other hidden, while cryptorchids have no testicles descended. The term cryptorchid literally translates to 'hidden testicle'. The lack of one or both testes must be investigated. If a cat has had both testes removed surgically, he is referred to as a castrate.

DIAGNOSING TESTICULAR PROBLEMS

Usually, a physical examination will reveal the problem. If necessary, X-ray or ultrasound examination may be used.

HOMEOPATHIC TREATMENT:
Thuja given orally. Your vet will advise you.

COST
Hormone treatment is relatively low cost, and surgical castration is quite a simple operation.

Testicular tumour

Underlying causes
The causes of cryptorchidism could include the testicles being hidden in the abdomen, or in the passage through the various layers of the abdominal muscles. They may even be outside the muscles, but under the skin; if this is the case, they can be easily located by feeling the area carefully. Anorchia is often due to congenital defects, or may be genetic in origin.

Treatment
Almost every cryptorchid has problems as he would be severely penalized or even disqualified in the show ring (depending on the rules pertaining) and is almost invariably sterile (or at the very least has an extremely low sperm count). It is strongly recommended that, unless your cat is destined only to be a pet, or you had already decided to have him castrated anyway, such animals should be avoided. Those who purchase such animals are strongly advised to have them surgically castrated at an early age.

🕲 COST
Could be high if there are any complications to the condition that require specialized or complicated surgery.

A tumour is a mass of cells which replicate at an extremely high rate.

Symptoms
Alopecia (see p.63), enlarged testicle(s), attractiveness to other male cats.

Underlying causes
Cryptorchids (see p.78) have a significantly higher risk than other intact cats of contracting testicular cancer. Mechanisms that bring on testicular cancer may be both hereditary and environmental.

Owner action
There is nothing that the owner of an affected cat can do.

Treatment
Castration followed by drugs is the routine treatment, and this is usually beneficial. The drugs help to kill the affected cells that may be left over after surgery.

DIAGNOSING TESTICULAR CANCER

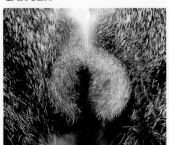

The vet will carry out a physical examination, and ask details of the cat's clinical history. The vet will want to know of any 'strange' behaviour or actions which you have noticed in your cat. 👁

URGENCY INDICATOR

Any cat showing any of the symptoms of testicular cancer should be taken for veterinary examination as soon as possible. Any delay allows the condition to advance and makes it more difficult to treat.

🕲 COST
Can be high. Several operations may be needed, and the drug therapy will be quite expensive, especially where the condition is not caught and treated in the early stages.

Queen problems

A queen has two ovaries, which produce the eggs. The ovaries are connected to the uterus by the fallopian tubes. The uterus is Y-shaped, and consists of two long horns. The eggs are fertilized in the fallopian tubes, which lead to the horns of the uterus where the eggs implant. The foetuses grow in the horns of the uterus throughout the gestation period or pregnancy. The wall of the uterus is made up of layers of smooth muscle called the myometrium. At the base of the uterus is the cervix, a muscular organ that closes the uterus except when the queen is mating or giving birth. The cervix is joined to the outside world by the vagina, and the vagina terminates as the vulva, or vaginal lips. Just inside the vagina is the 'vestibule', a chamber with extremely strong muscles in its wall. It is these muscles that help 'tie' the tom and queen during mating.

- **Pro-oestrus** The beginning of heat in the queen, when the vulva swells and there is a blood-stained discharge. This stage lasts two or three days, and toms will be very attracted by the queen, but she will not allow them to mate her.
- **Oestrus** The period when the queen will accept a mating from a tom. She may call incessantly, in an effort to attract tom cats. She will roll about and rub against furniture and other solid objects. The vulva is extremely enlarged and swollen, and the discharge is straw-coloured. This phase lasts three to five days. About two days after oestrus begins, ovulation occurs.
- **Interoestrus** Occurs only in the unmated queen or in a queen who has been mated but has not conceived. The signs of oestrus will fade and the queen is not receptive to the advances of toms. This stage lasts between three and 14 days. After interoestrus the queen's cycle returns to pro-oestrus then oestrus, except in the winter months (see below).
- **Anoestrus** The period between cycles. In queens, it occurs in the winter months when she is sexually inactive.

Most queens reach puberty at between six and nine months, but this depends entirely upon the daylength. A queen born in the winter may not begin to cycle until she is 12 months old. If a queen has not had a season by the time she is 18 months old, then veterinary advice should be sought.

If you do not intend to breed from a queen, there are many advantages to having her spayed (neutered or sterilized) when she is young, as she will not then suffer from diseases of the ovaries or uterus, since they are removed in the operation. You also do not run the risk of unwanted pregnancies.

Pseudo pregnancy

Often it is difficult to tell the difference between a pseudo pregnancy and the real thing, as the queen's abdomen will swell in each case.

False or phantom pregnancy. Pseudo pregnancies are quite natural, and may occur in a queen that has failed to conceive in a given oestrus. The effects differ with different queens.

Symptoms

In some cases of pseudo pregnancy, the owner may not notice any difference in either the queen's physical or mental condition. In other queens, the pseudo pregnancy may mean that the cat's abdomen swells, her mammary glands (teats) fill with milk, and her mental attitude will change. She will spend much time nest-building, she will cry and be reluctant to take any exercise, and may even go through the pushing and thrusting of an actual birth. Many such queens will form emotional attachments to inanimate objects, particularly their toys, and some have 'invisible' kittens. The queen's territorial and maternal aggression will show, as she protects her invisible litter, and this can be extremely upsetting for the owner of the queen. Many of the queens that exhibit symptoms of pseudo pregnancy will show more marked symptoms season after season throughout their life.

DIAGNOSING PSEUDO PREGNANCY

The vet will examine the queen, to ensure that she is not actually pregnant.

Underlying causes

This is usually due to a non-fertile mating, that is being mated with a tom that cannot produce viable sperm.

Owner action

The queen should not be allowed toys and similar objects to play with.

Treatment

In mild cases, most vets will recommend that the queen is left to go through the phase on her own. In severe cases, the vet may recommend that the queen is given hormone treatment.

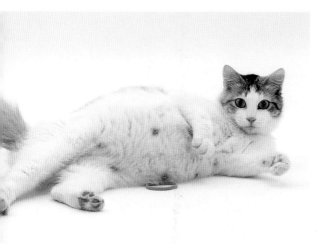

⊙ Cost

Should be quite low as normally 'treatment' consists of allowing the queen to go through the pseudo pregnancy. Hormone treatment is also relatively low cost.

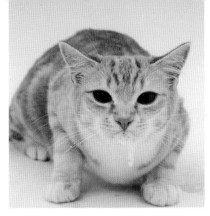

Misalliance

A mating that was not intended.

Owner action

To prevent misalliance occurring, take care to ensure that you do not let your cat out when she is in season.

Treatment

The vet will administer an injection of hormones, which will override the effects of the queen's own hormones, making her body believe that she is not pregnant, and causing oestrus to begin again. Vets do not like to give such injections as a matter of course, since they can sometimes have very serious side effects, including the development of pyometra (see p.84). Prevention is always better than cure, and so all queens in season, and therefore receptive to the attentions of a male cat, should be kept out of trouble or temptation.

Eclampsia

'Milk fever' or lactation tetany (the paralysis of milk production in the dam's teats), seen after kittening.

Symptoms

An affected queen will be anxious and will shy away from light. She may totally ignore her kittens, often wandering away from them, salivate profusely and be extremely uncoordinated. The queen's body temperature will rise from 39°C to 41°C (102°F to 106°F) or even higher, her heart rate will increase, and she will have convulsions.

Underlying causes

Eclampsia is usually due to the cat's diet

Symptoms of 'milk fever' include salivating. Increasing the amount of calcium in your cat's diet can help counter eclampsia.

being low in calcium. It can occur up to 21 days after kittening, although very rarely it can occur just prior to kittening.

Owner action

As this is such an extremely serious condition, veterinary treatment must be sought immediately, and there is nothing that the owner can do.

Treatment

The vet will treat the condition with calcium and glucose, which may be delivered via intraperitoneal injections (injections into the abdomen) or an intravenous drip. The results really are spectacular, as the queen can recover in just a few minutes.

DIAGNOSING ECLAMPSIA

The vet will physically examine the queen.

Nymphomania

Queens with increased sexual drive or unusual oestrus cycles.

Symptoms
While this term may be used for queens who have increased sexual drive (libido), it is also used to describe queens who have more oestruses than normal, where pro-oestrus (the beginning stage of oestrus) is abnormally long, and those queens which show more than normal interest in male cats.

Underlying causes
It is thought that the condition is caused by enlarged ovarian follicles (cavities in the ovary) producing too much oestrogen (a female sex hormone).

Owner action
Contact the vet for advice. If the queen's sex drive is increased, she should be kept indoors at all times.

URGENCY INDICATOR

This condition is best treated as soon as possible to prevent any harmful and long-term side effects as a result of too much oestrogen being produced in the queen's body.

DIAGNOSING NYMPHOMANIA

Where the ovarian follicles are enlarged, the vet will carry out physical, X-ray or ultrasonic examinations.

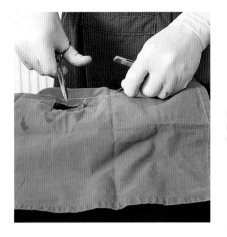

Having your cat spayed is the best treatment for nymphomania.

Treatment
In chronic cases where the queen will not be used for breeding purposes, spaying is the best treatment. In other cases hormone injections will probably work.

🕐 COST
Normal treatment is low cost. Surgical spaying is a relatively simple operation.

Metritis

Infection of the inner lining of the uterus, the endometrium, which occurs immediately after kittening.

Symptoms
Include a foul-smelling discharge from the queen's vulva, lack of appetite, reduced milk production, and vomiting.

Underlying causes
This condition is caused by a bacterial infection.

Treatment
Treatment will consist of antibiotics, and the queen may be given supportive drugs to help her fight the condition.

DIAGNOSING METRITIS

Physical examination, often supported by analysis of the discharge.

URGENCY INDICATOR

A vet must be consulted immediately as this condition is potentially life-threatening.

🕐 COST
If caught early enough, costs will be low. Any complications will add to the cost of treatment.

Vaginal prolapse or hyperplasia

When the lining of the vagina prolapses through the vulva.

Symptoms

In older, entire queens, who have had many oestrus cycles, the lining of the vagina may protrude through the vulva: it will be seen as a red, swollen mass that may be as big as a large chicken egg.

DIAGNOSING HYPERPLASIA

Physical examination by a vet. ◉

Underlying causes

The problem usually occurs after kittening, and is often a result of wear and tear.

Owner action

Keep the queen calm, and contact the vet.

Treatment

The condition often requires surgery. Where the problem recurs regularly, spaying is the best course of action.

URGENCY INDICATOR

Seek immediate veterinary treatment for the affected queen. If the protruding lining becomes damaged, it is very easy for the queen to suffer massive blood loss.

◔ **COST**

The surgery required can often be quite complicated, so the costs may well be high.

This condition is most likely to occur after your cat has given birth.

Pyometra

Infection of the queen's uterus. This condition is quite rare in cats.

Symptoms

The most obvious and earliest symptom of pyometra is an increased thirst, leading to increased drinking, leading in turn to increased urination.
Other symptoms may include:
- *a poor quality coat*
- *vomiting*
- *lethargy and a general reluctance to take any exercise*
- *reluctance to eat or even anorexia*
- *a discharge of mucus from the vulva after the season has finished and*
- *excessive licking of the vulva*

URGENCY INDICATOR

A severe case of pyometra can be life-threatening, so you should watch out for any of the symptoms listed above, which may appear within a few weeks of the queen's oestrus. If your queen is exhibiting any of these symptoms, you should seek veterinary advice as soon as possible.

DIAGNOSING PYOMETRA

Although this is not a common problem in queens, the vet will recognize the signs of pyometra. Occasionally, the vet may use X-ray and ultrasound examinations to confirm the diagnosis, or may take samples of any discharge from the vulva for laboratory analysis. ◉

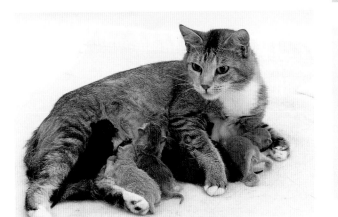

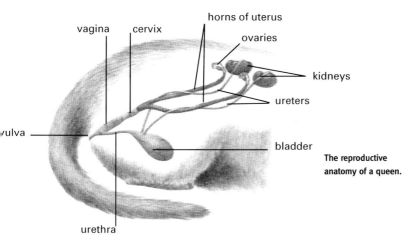

The reproductive anatomy of a queen.

Underlying causes

Pyometra is caused by bacteria, probably from the queen's urinary system, and it is believed that the higher than normal hormone levels in the queen during oestrus may help promote the growth of the bacteria. The infection causes the uterus to swell and fill with pus, and in some cases, the uterus can reach almost gigantic proportions. Once the condition present there, it will get progressively worse with every season that the queen has. Spayed queens cannot develop pyometra.

Owner action

Seek veterinary advice if you see any of the symptoms of pyometra.

Treatment

The treatment for pyometra is for the queen to be spayed as soon as possible, unless she is too ill for the operation. If this is the case, the vet will treat the queen with antibiotics and maybe an intravenous drip, until she is well enough for the operation.

COST
Surgery will be
involved, and in
severe cases
intensive care will be
needed, so costs
could be quite high.

Vaginitis

Infection of the vagina leading to inflammation.

Symptoms

A thick, creamy discharge from the lips of the vulva. The queen will probably spend much time licking her vulva to remove this discharge.

DIAGNOSING VAGINITIS

The vet will take smears from the lining of the vagina. This sample is cultured in a laboratory and the organisms responsible for the infection are identified.

Underlying causes

Vaginitis is caused by harmful bacteria or the herpes virus.

Owner action

Keep the queen calm and quiet and consult the vet.

Treatment

A course of antibiotics. These should be taken as directed, and the course must be completed.

URGENCY INDICATOR

Seek veterinary treatment within 24 hours otherwise the condition will become acute and will be more difficult to treat.

COST
Modern antibiotics
are effective and
cost relatively little.

Mastitis

If the queen is
suffering from
mastitis, the
amount of milk
available for her
litter will be less
than is needed. It
is important that
you contact the
vet as soon as
the condition is
noticed, as
occasionally if it
is not treated,
mastitis can lead
to quite severe
problems for the
affected queen.

When a nursing queen
is suffering from
mastitis, it may well be
necessary to hand feed
the kittens to ensure
their health.

⏁ **COST**

Low, especially if
caught in the early
stages of the
condition.

Inflammation of the queen's mammary
glands during lactation (the production of
milk to feed a litter).

Symptoms

*Mastitis results in hard teats that feel
hot to the touch; any milk produced by
an infected teat may be bloodstained
and/or look abnormal. The affected
queen will be 'off colour'; she will have
little or no appetite, and may vomit.*

DIAGNOSING MASTITIS

Mastitis can be diagnosed by
physical examination by a vet. 👁

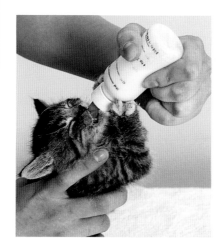

RELATED CONDITIONS
WHICH MAY PRODUCE
SIMILAR SYMPTOMS

A queen suffering a pseudo pregnancy
(see p.81) may also develop
mastitis. *ⓘ*

Underlying causes

Mastitis is caused by bacterial infection by
streptococci bacteria.

Owner action

While any teat is not functioning properly, it
will be necessary to check the litter even
more carefully than usual to ensure that
they are getting enough milk. If there are
several teats affected by mastitis, and so
not delivering enough – or even any – milk,
it may be necessary to hand rear one or
more kittens.

To help prevent mastitis, wipe the
queen's abdomen clean on a regular basis,
preferably using a mild anti-bacterial
cleaner which the vet will recommend. The
kittens should also be encouraged to use
all teats evenly, although this may not be
possible where the litter is very small. In
such cases, careful hand stripping of the
milk in the unused teats may be called for.
The vet will demonstrate how to do this;
throughout hand stripping, ensure that you
maintain the highest degree of personal
hygiene, and wash your hands before and
after the procedure; it is also advisable to
wash your hands between teats to avoid
transferring the infection.

Treatment

Antibiotics will be prescribed. Often, carefully stripping out the milk by hand will be
necessary (see above), and the queen will
get some relief from having the affected
mammary gland(s) bathed in warm water.
In very rare cases, lancing or surgery may
be necessary. Where proper treatment is
sought and given, most cases of mastitis
will clear up within 36–48 hours.

Mammary cancer

Cancer of the breast. Extremely common in unspayed queens, almost half of all mammary tumours are malignant (progressively worsening and invariably fatal if left untreated).

Symptoms
Lumps in the queen's mammary glands ('teats').

If any lumps are found in a queen's teat, she should be given a full examination by a vet. The earlier a tumour is found and treatment is begun, the better the prognosis for the cat.

🄯 COST
As treatment is often complicated and long-term, costs can be quite high.

DIAGNOSING MAMMARY CANCER

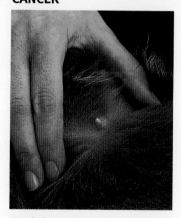

A typical mammary tumour will appear as a well-defined lump in the queen's teat. It may only be the size of a pea when first noticed, but the lump will increase in size as the queen comes into oestrus.

To identify whether the problem is a tumour, the vet may use many types of examination, including physical, X-ray, ultrasound and blood tests. Once a tumour is confirmed, further tests will be given to identify the tumour's type, size, exact location and the degree to which it may have spread. As this is such a specialized area, the vet may refer you to a specialist vet.

Underlying causes
Not entirely known, but the condition is believed to be linked with hormone in many cases.

Owner action
It is worthwhile examining your queen's teats for lumps on a regular basis, as it is always better to treat this (and any other ailment) in its early stages.

Treatment
The treatment for mammary tumours may include surgery (cutting out or reducing the tumour), chemotherapy (the use of drugs to kill or shrink the tumour), radiotherapy (the use of ionizing radiation to kill the tumour cells, often used in conjunction with surgery), or hyperthermia. The latter involves the application of extremely high temperatures to a tumour, via ultrasound or electromagnetic radiation.

As veterinary science advances, more and more is discovered about tumours, and how to successfully treat them. Many tumours that at one stage were felt to be beyond treatment are now being successfully treated, leading to improvement in the cat's quality of life, and a longer life.

Mammary cancers may not be obvious to the eye, and so it is important that you check your cat regularly.

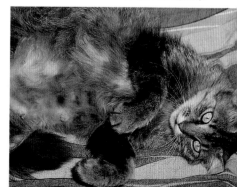

Elderly cat problems

As veterinary science advances, coupled with similar advances in the production of cat foods, cats are living longer and healthier lives. The average life span of a cat is about 14 years, and some cats can live for over 20 years. Good husbandry, including good nutrition, checking a kitten's parents for hereditary diseases, and good medical care, can all increase both the quality and length of a cat's life. However, old age brings with it wear and tear on the body and its organs, and this causes certain physical and behavioural changes and ailments.

Even though a young cat will sleep for many hours of the day, an elderly cat will require even more rest, and will sleep very deeply. Many cats will get grey hairs, although this greying may start well before the age at which the cat could be described as elderly. An elderly cat may not wish to exercise anywhere near as much as she used to, and she should not be subjected to extremes of temperature, so do not put your cat out on a cold night, and do not let her sleep on a cold concrete floor.

An elderly cat's appetite may change, and her nutritional requirements will alter, and vitamin and/or mineral supplements may be necessary. Always consult the vet before you give any supplement to your cat.

Many problems and medical conditions which, while the cat was young, were considered minor and of little consequence, may become more serious as the cat ages. The following are some of the problems and conditions which are particularly common in older cats.

Tooth decay

**If your cat's teeth become diseased,
she may show a reluctance to eat her
food, particularly if the food is hard
(such as biscuits). Examination of her
teeth may reveal obvious 'bad' (decayed)
teeth, or halitosis (bad breath – see
p.21). A veterinary examination will
reveal whether any treatment can be
given, which will improve the cat's
quality of life.**

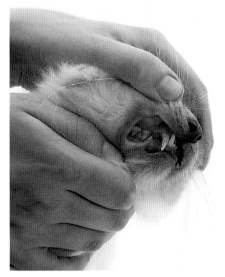

Although many cats
will object to it, it is
good practice to check
your cat's teeth at
regular intervals in
order to pick up on any
tooth problems in their
early stages.

Obesity

URGENCY INDICATOR

The sooner the cat loses the weight the better, although ideally you should not allow your cat to become overweight in the first place.

Many older cats become overweight, and this is a major cause of many potentially life-threatening diseases.

Symptoms

A cat that has too much fat for its day-to-day activities will store the fat under it skin. In cases of severe obesity this will result in rolls of skin and fat.

DIAGNOSING OBESITY

It is possible to obtain tables giving the ideal weight ranges for different breeds, but most vets will not adhere to them too firmly, as they are only a guide. Each cat is an individual, and needs to be treated as such. Common sense will guide you as to whether your cat has a weight problem, and the vet will advise you on how best to tackle the situation.

Underlying causes

As she gets older, and no longer wishes to take as much exercise as she once did, your cat may put on weight; this extra weight will make her more prone to many diseases, including heart problems.

Owner action

If your cat is overweight, you will need to adjust her diet. The answer is not just to reduce the amount of food that you feed her, as many cats then address their constant hunger by scavenging, even if they never did this in their earlier years. The best method of ensuring your cat loses weight is to change her diet for one of the many low-calorie diets specifically produced by food manufacturers for elderly cats. These foods may also help prevent or alleviate some of the problems that may affect older cats. Always consult the vet before drastically changing your cat's diet. Many vets have a trained dietary adviser.

If you feed a mix of meat (either tinned or fresh) and biscuit, the you should change the biscuits for a low-calorie type to reduce the total amount of calories that your cat ingests each day. The biscuits, in whole or in part, can also be substituted with cooked vegetables to help reduce the weight of your cat.

WARNING: OBESITY IS VERY DANGEROUS TO A CAT OF ANY AGE.

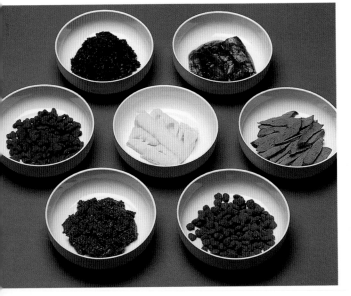

Ensuring your cat has a healthy diet from an early age will help prevent obesity in later life.

Coat problems

A cat's coat changes as time passes, and many of the 'problems' associated with the cat's coat are an inevitable part of the ageing process.

Symptoms

The cat's coat may become greasier or drier, and tends to become matted and 'tatty' very easily. Also, as the cat ages she may have longer claws than normal, due to her getting less exercise, which would normally wear the claws down.

DIAGNOSING COAT PROBLEMS

There could be several reasons for your cat's condition, so the vet will need to carry out a physical examination and in some cases blood samples may also be taken and tested.

For many coat problems, your vet may prescribe a special shampoo with which to wash the affected cat at specific intervals.

Underlying causes

As a cat gets older, the texture and character of her coat will change. The cause is often linked to an increase in thyroid hormones in the cat's body, a normal consequence of the ageing process.

Owner action

To keep the coat in good condition, bath and groom your cat at more regular intervals, and also check her claws, clipping them as and when necessary. When clipping a cat's claws, it is essential that you use the correct clippers: that is, those designed especially for the task, and get advice from the vet on how to use them in the proper way.

It may be advantageous with some cats to have the coat clipped out; this will be extremely beneficial to long-haired cats whose coats are liable to become matted.

Treatment

Treatment will vary depending on the underlying causes of the coat condition, but is usually based on diet. If you are feeding your cat a diet high in fats, this will tend to make the coat greasy.

URGENCY INDICATOR

This condition will irritate your cat, and this irritation will lead to a further deterioration in her condition, so you should consult the vet.

🔄 COST

If the treatment consists only of changing the diet, costs will be low, but as coat problems may be a symptom of more serious conditions, costs can vary greatly.

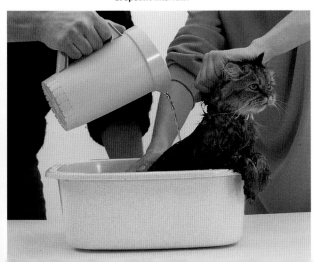

RELATED CONDITIONS WHICH MAY PRODUCE SIMILAR SYMPTOMS

Roundworm infestation, renal failure (see p.38), diabetes mellitus (see p.23) and hyperthyroidism.

Senility

The mental deterioration of an animal due (usually) to old age.

Symptoms

As your cat reaches old age, you will notice that on some days she will seem to behave perfectly normally, but on other days she may be restless and disorientated. Often, a cat suffering from senility will seem to want to spend more time in the company of her owner, and demand more attention from members of the human family.

Underlying causes

Senility is almost always due to the normal ageing process, whereby damaged cells, in this case in the brain, are no longer being replaced as they were before.

Owner action

It is important for the human family to provide plenty of tender, loving care and understanding to an elderly cat.

Treatment

There is no cure for senility, but it may be possible to administer drugs that will improve your cat's quality of life, for example by helping to control incontinence. Considerate nursing will help improve the cat's quality of life.

URGENCY INDICATOR

If your cat shows these symptoms, you should take her to the vet for examination.

◔ **COST**

Drugs may be provided for the problems associated with senility, and the cost will depend on the extent and nature of these other problems.

DIAGNOSING SENILITY

The vet will test for a lower than normal response to stimuli and look for any signs of disorientation.

Incontinence

Incontinence may be urinary (see p.37), fecal or both.

Symptoms

A complete or partial inability to control urination and/or defecation, leading to your cat having 'accidents', often extremely frequently.

URGENCY INDICATOR

This condition is upsetting for all concerned. It is therefore best to consult a vet as soon as the problem becomes apparent.

DIAGNOSING CAUSES OF INCONTINENCE

In elderly cats, the most common (and likely) cause of incontinence will be lack of muscle tone (to control urination or defecation).

Underlying causes

As the cat ages, muscles become inefficient, and this can lead to incontinence. Fecal incontinence may be caused by a flabby anal sphincter muscle (the ring of muscle that opens the anus to the outside). Cystitis (see p.36) is the most common cause in queens, although faulty or 'lazy' urethral valves may also be the cause. These control the flow of urine, and are muscles situated around the urethra. In 'lazy' valves, the muscles do not seal the urethra off properly, or, in some cases, do not seal it off at all. Any such problem should be investigated by the vet.

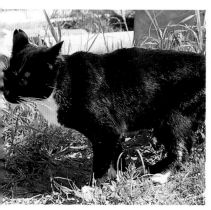

Urinary and fecal incontinence in elderly cats is usually due to a lack of muscle tone.

In many cases, wet beds are simply the result of the cat feeling unable or unwilling to make the effort to get up. Arthritis (see p.44) is a major cause of an elderly cat lacking the will to move.

Owner action

There is very little the owner can do, except to allow the cat the opportunity to relieve herself by allowing her out last thing at night, or before she is confined for any reason.

Treatment

Very little can be done to treat incontinence caused by the ageing process, although some drugs may alleviate the problem slightly.

 COST
Little treatment is possible.

Liver failure

The liver is one of the main organs of the cat's body. It has many complex roles, including helping the kidneys remove waste products from the cat's body, the production of proteins involved in blood clotting, the processing and storing of fats and carbohydrates, production of bile (necessary for digestion), and the general purification of the blood. Any major problems with the liver will have serious effects on the cat.

Symptoms

Symptoms can be very difficult to detect, particularly in the early stages of this condition. They may include the cat going off her food, weight loss, vomiting, diarrhoea or general lack of condition in the cat. Jaundice may be seen in the mucous membranes.

DIAGNOSING LIVER FAILURE

The vet will do blood and urine tests to look for any abnormalities, and may need to take X-rays and carry out ultrasound examinations to see any physical changes.

Underlying causes

Long-term inflammation of the liver, cancer, or problems with the bile duct (the tube down which bile passes) can all be causes of liver failure.

Owner action

There is nothing that the owner can do apart from contacting the vet as soon as possible.

Treatment

Unfortunately, there is often very little that can be done for a cat suffering from chronic liver failure, as the problem will not become apparent until it has become so serious that the cat is beyond treatment.

URGENCY INDICATOR

If your cat is showing any symptoms of liver problems it is important to have her examined by a vet as soon as possible.

COST
As there is no treatment available, there will be no costs.

Other medical disorders

This chapter gives information on a range of other disorders that may affect your cat, and which cannot easily be categorized.

Behaviour problems

Throughout a cat's life, her behaviour will change in small ways. It is wise to make a note of any behavioural changes, and if they persist, you should seek advice from the vet. If you are concerned about any aspect of your cat's behaviour, do not hesitate to contact the vet, as many problems are far easier to treat if they are caught early. If you ignore a problem it may develop into a major, possibly life-threatening, condition.

Some common changes in behaviour are:
Insatiable appetite: Especially when this is accompanied by weight loss, the cat may have a problem with her pancreas or be suffering from a large infestation of worms. The pancreas is responsible for the secretion of pancreatic enzymes, which are essential for digestion.
Loss of appetite: This may be due to mouth ulcers, congestion of the nose, an infectious disease or a metabolic disease (one that affects the body's ability to properly digest and utilize food).
Pica: A craving for unnatural foods, which may result from a poor diet. Affected cats may eat their own droppings, the faeces of farm animals, such as cows or horses, or even stones, rocks and pebbles. A 'favourite' material for cats to chew is wool. Where a cat eats fecal matter, this is known as coprophagy.
Polydipsia: Excessive thirst. The cause may be dietary or a disease such as diabetes mellitus (see p.24).
Pacing, panting, incessant mewing, scratching at the floor or bedding: These are all signs of restlessness in a cat. They may indicate that the cat feels uncomfortable, or is in pain; that the room temperature is too hot or too cold; that she needs to go to the toilet; that she is lonely or that she is bored. If your cat has had dressings put on an injury or wound, these may be too tight, and this will also make the cat feel restless. Depending upon the cause, steps should always be taken to alleviate a cat's distress if at all possible.

Physiological problems

You may also observe physiological changes in your cat.

Some common physiological problems include:

Aural discharge: Discharge from the ears, possibly due to an infection, or an injury.

Changes in the colour of the cat's mucous membranes: The best way to see this is to examine the inside of the cat's mouth, particularly her gums. Pale gums may indicate anaemia (see p.18), haemorrhage or heart problems (see p.15 and 17). Gums that appear slightly blue (cyanosis) may indicate a breathing problem. Gums that appear to have a yellow tinge (jaundice) may indicate that the cat has liver problems (see p.93), or leptospirosis, a highly infectious disease caused by bacteria.

● **Constipation** (see p.32).

● **Diarrhoea** (see p.30). To help the vet identify the cause of diarrhoea, which is a symptom of many different conditions, you should try to note the frequency, colour, smell and consistency of the motions passed by your cat.

● **Nasal discharge**: Discharge from the nose, usually caused by an infection, but may be due to a foreign body.

● **Ocular discharge**: Discharge from the eye(s), usually caused by infection, but may be due to a foreign body.

● **Polyuria**. The production of large amounts of urine, possibly due to damaged or infected kidneys.

● **Vaginal discharge**: Caused by a bacterial infection or the herpes virus.

● **Vomiting** (see p.28). To help the vet identify the cause of this symptom, the frequency and volume of vomit should be noted, as should the presence of blood or mucus in the vomit.

Feline T-lymphotropic lentivirus (FTLV) Also known as feline immunodeficiency virus (FIV)

A viral infection that affects the RNA (ribonucleic acid) that is involved in the manufacture of proteins within the cat's cells. It prevents the body's immuno-defence system from fighting off infections.

Symptoms

This virus allows many infections to become established in the affected cat but has no symptoms as such.

DIAGNOSING FTLV

Laboratory analysis of a blood sample.

Underlying causes

The virus multiplies in the white cells in the cat's blood, and is often transmitted via cat bites.

Owner action

Cats suspected of suffering an FTLV infection must be taken to the vet. Infected cats will suffer chronic, long-term illnesses, weight loss etc. as a result of the infections caused by the lack of immuno-response.

Treatment

There is currently no treatment available for a cat infected with FTLV, and euthanasia is usually recommended.

RELATED CONDITIONS WHICH MAY PRODUCE SIMILAR SYMPTOMS

This virus is closely related to the FeLV virus (see p.96) and may produce similar secondary symptoms. ⓘ

URGENCY INDICATOR

Severely affected cats will suffer from many infections, so veterinary treatment must be sought urgently.

 COST
The cost will be the cost of treating the associated illnesses.

Feline leukaemia virus (FeLV)

A viral infection that affects the cat's immuno-response system.

Symptoms

Lethargy, high temperature, lack of appetite and enlarged lymph nodes.

DIAGNOSING FɛLV

Laboratory analysis of a blood sample.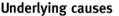

 COST

There is currently no treatment for this condition, although costs may be incurred if any other conditions brought on by the FeLV infection need to be treated.

FeLV is often passed between cats during mating, as the virus is contained in the body fluids of the infected animal.

Underlying causes

The viral infection prevents the cat's immuno-response system from functioning adequately: that is, the body cannot fight off infections of any kind. The condition is spread mainly by matings and also via bite wounds as the virus is contained in the cat's body fluids, which include saliva, blood and semen.

Owner action

There is a vaccine available for this condition, and owners are recommended to have their cat vaccinated on a regular basis. If your cat is diagnosed as having FeLV, you must carefully consider what this means for the cat's future, and discuss the possibilities with your vet. Some owners prefer not to risk their cat infecting others, so choose to have the infected cat put to sleep.

Treatment

There is no cure for FeLV. Many cats infected with the disease will make a reasonable recovery naturally, but will then become carriers, spreading the condition to all other cats with which they come into contact. If you have more than one cat in your home, the vet may recommend that the infected cat is put to sleep in order to prevent the infection spreading to other cats. If you have just one cat, you must never allow her to go outside, where she may come into contact with, and therefore infect, other cats in your neighbourhood.

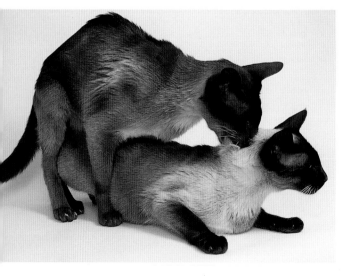

RELATED CONDITIONS WHICH MAY PRODUCE SIMILAR SYMPTOMS

FTLV (see p.95).

Toxoplasmosis

Infection by an endoparasite, *Toxoplasma gondii*. This is a very small parasite that lives in the cells lining the cat's intestines.

Symptoms

Most of the cats infected with this extremely common condition never show any symptoms. Cats suffering a severe toxoplasmosis infection may have any or all of the following symptoms
- *weight loss*
- *loss of appetite*
- *fever*
- *breathing difficulties and*
- *diarrhoea*

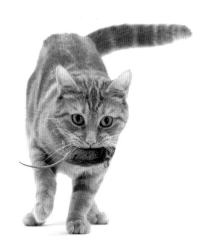

Most cats contract toxoplasmosis from eating infected wild mice.

DIAGNOSING TOXOPLASMOSIS

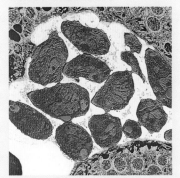

Laboratory analysis of feces and/or blood.

 COST

If caught early, costs will be low. However, severe infection can lead to dangerous conditions, so costs will escalate.

Underlying causes

Your cat may become infected by the eggs of the endoparasite by eating wild mice or uncooked infected meat.

Owner action

Humans are an intermediate host for this parasite. An intermediate host is the animal in which the parasite undergoes a stage in its development. Pregnant women can suffer serious medical problems that may threaten their unborn child if they become infected. This infection can be caused by eating undercooked infected meat, or by handling the feces of infected cats (for example, in litter trays). Ensuring that your cat is adequately and regularly treated for endoparasites will greatly reduce the risk of human members of the family becoming infected. It is vitally important that you always take great care over your personal hygiene when handling any cat, and especially when emptying and cleaning soiled litter trays, when you should wear gloves.

Treatment

The vet will prescribe a suitable drug to kill the organism responsible for the infection.

Epilepsy

Epilepsy is a disturbance in the body's nervous system which results in the cat twitching quite violently. It is a relatively rare condition in cats.

Symptoms

Regular, repeated convulsions or 'fits', due to violent contractions of muscles, a result of the abnormal electrical activity of the brain. If these seizures are not treated, they will recur at shorter and shorter intervals, eventually leading to status epilepticus, which is a state of continuous seizures.

Never take a cat that is fitting to the vet in a carry box, as she may well cause more injury to herself.

There are three phases to seizures;
1 The aura – lasting from a couple of minutes to several days. During this phase, the cat appears agitated and anxious.
2 The ictus – the cat passes into unconsciousness. Her eyes will be staring, and her legs rigid, and this is quickly followed by 'jaw-champing' and fast paddling actions of the legs. Within a few minutes of this, the cat's breathing will become extremely strenuous.
3 The post-ictal phase – the cat's convulsive movements will stop, and her muscles relax. At the same time, her breathing will return to normal, and the cat will regain consciousness. When she has come around, she will appear confused and dazed for up to two days. During this recovery period, the cat may eat far more than normal, mew and cry more, and spend a great deal of time pacing around.

If a cat suffers partial seizures, which only affect one part of the body, the symptoms may include rapid side-to-side movement of the head, spasms in the legs (sometimes only one leg is affected), or unusual behaviour, such as aggression or even screaming for no apparent reason.

☻ COST

Low to medium, depending on the underlying causes. Anticonvulsant drugs are one of the cheaper treatments.

DIAGNOSING EPILEPSY

The vet may have to carry out physical and neurological examinations, a brain scan, blood and urine tests and spinal fluid tests in order to reach an accurate diagnosis.

Cancers or lymphomas

Underlying causes

Epilepsy results from disturbances in the cat's central nervous system, resulting from electrical abnormalities in the brain. There are many possible causes of fitting and epilepsy, including infections (either viral or bacterial), head injuries, brain tumours, hypocalcaemia (low levels of calcium in the cat's blood), hypoglycaemia (abnormally low levels of sugar in the cat's blood), renal (kidney) disease, liver disease or poisoning.

If a cat is epileptic, she will probably suffer her first seizure between the ages of one and three years. In young cats and kittens, seizures may be a symptom of an infection.

Owner action

If your cat is fitting, do not touch her, but move any objects around her on which she could injure herself. Keep quiet and, if possible, darken the area. As she comes out of her fit, speak calmly and quietly to your cat to reassure and comfort her. *Never* place a cat that is having a fit in your car and drive her to the veterinary practice; wait until she has recovered and then take her, ensuring that you drive steadily, and do not further upset her. In some cases, it may be necessary for the cat to be kept where she is, and the vet will attend her at home.

Treatment

The root cause of the problem will need to be identified before the epilepsy can be treated. Anticonvulsant drugs may be prescribed by the vet, but only if the fitting is regular and persistent.

A term given to a group of diseases. It refers to malignant tumours and leukaemia, and is quite common in cats. A tumour is an abnormal swelling, which may be malignant (progressively worsening and resulting in death if left untreated) or benign.

Symptoms

These will depend on the type of the cancer, its location, size and how it is interfering with other parts of the cat's body. Many cancers are not detectable by the owner until they are in an advanced state.

DIAGNOSING CANCER

The vet will carry out physical, X-ray and ultrasound examinations, blood tests and internal examinations (perhaps using an endoscope).

Underlying causes

There are many factors that can cause cancer, both environmental and congenital (present from birth).

Owner action

There is nothing that an owner of a cat affected by cancer can do.

Treatment

Treatment is more likely to be successful if the cancer is caught at an early stage. Treatments vary according to the cause, severity and position of the cancer.

In chemotherapy, cytotoxic drugs are used. These are designed to kill the cells in the cancer, and are used either on their own, or following surgery, to ensure that no malignant cells remain in the cat's body.

URGENCY INDICATOR

If you suspect that your cat has any form of cancer, you must seek advice from the vet as soon as possible.

COST

The cost of treatment for some cancers can be extremely high, as the treatment may be prolonged and complicated.

Cushing's disease

Technically known as hyperadrenocorticalism, Cushing's disease occurs when the cat's adrenal glands produce excessive amounts of cortisol, a steroid hormone. There are two adrenal glands, situated near the kidneys. They produce hormones that help the body to meet emergencies by increasing the blood glucose level and/or increasing the heart rate.

Symptoms

Cats affected by Cushing's disease may show the following symptoms:
- *alopecia on the flanks (see p.63)*
- *coat colour changes*
- *muscle wasting and general debilitation*
- *polydipsia (an excessive thirst)*
- *polyuria (production of large amounts of urine) and*
- *swelling of the abdomen (due to an enlarged liver and fluid retention)*

DIAGNOSING CUSHING'S DISEASE

The vet will carry out hormone tests, which will determine if Cushing's disease is present and also reveal the cause of the problem, and therefore the treatment.

Underlying causes

The cause of Cushing's disease is a tumour of the pituitary gland, or, less commonly, an adrenal gland tumour. A pituitary tumour will lead to excessive amounts of adrenocorticotrophic hormone, which in turn will stimulate the adrenal gland to produce excess cortisol.

Owner action

There is nothing that an owner of a cat affected by Cushing's disease can do.

Treatment

Where the problem is caused by an adrenal tumour, the affected gland may be surgically removed. Where the problem is in the pituitary gland, drug treatment (mitotane) will be given by mouth; this drug is given with food, and the person giving the drug must take care to wear gloves while handling it. The vet will need to monitor the affected cat to determine the actual dosage of the drug needed to achieve the target of treating the polydipsia, that is – reducing the cat's water intake.

Euthanasia

There comes a time when having your cat put painlessly to sleep is the kindest treatment. Reaching that decision can be extremely distressing for the owner and other people concerned, but the welfare and happiness of the cat must be given priority at all times. Owners all too often postpone the inevitable, mainly because they cannot bear the thought of being parted from their beloved pet. Whilst this is perfectly understandable, it is also unfair on the cat.

Even though it may be the most humane course of action, reaching the decision to put your cat to sleep will be distressing for the owner and all those concerned.

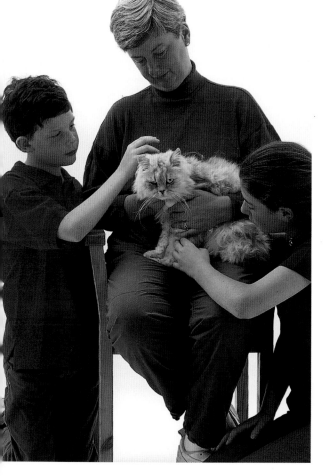

Euthanasia is carried out by your vet administering a lethal dose of barbiturates via an injection into the cat's veins. The process is entirely painless for the cat.

The owner always makes the final decision to end a pet's life, but the decision should be based on information and advice from the vet. Never be afraid to ask the vet for details of the condition, what the future may hold for the cat if she is not put to sleep, and the physical and mental state of your cat. You will never be rushed to make this decision, and you may wish to discuss it with other members of your family. Make sure you explain to everyone what is going to happen to your cat, especially where children are involved, so that no one is under any illusions.

Once the decision has been made, you should spend a little time considering the practicalities. You may wish to have you cat's body cremated or buried, and so will need to make these arrangements before taking your cat on her final visit to the veterinary practice. Many vets will allow the cat's body to remain at the practice until collected by the pet funeral service, and this may help you to cope with your grief over the loss of a loved one. Do not worry about crying in the surgery; this is perfectly normal and no one will think any the less of you for this action. It often helps to spend a few minutes alone with your cat prior to euthanasia and afterwards, and your vet will respect your wishes.

Feelings of sadness, anger and guilt are quite normal for the owner of any animal that has been put to sleep. Your vet may be able to offer you counselling. One of the best ways to get over the death of a beloved pet is to be sure that you have acted at all times in the best interests of your cat, and that she has had a good, happy life with you.

Accidents and emergencies

There are many cases where a knowledge of first aid can be useful, and some where it is essential. Accidents happen when we least expect them to, so it is sensible to be prepared to carry out first aid. Emergency situations require immediate action, and if you are familiar with first aid practice you will be able to limit the injuries sustained by your cat, and in some cases, you may even save her life.

All first aid principles are the same, regardless of whether you are dealing with a person or an animal, and everyone should have a basic training in the subject. This will give you confidence and this confidence, will help you to keep calm in an emergency situation – vital where the cat's life is, quite literally, in your hands until a trained practitioner can take over from you. First aid organizations throughout the world run courses, and going on such a course may help you to save a life. It is important to practice relevant procedures *before* you encounter an emergency. Most vets will help with this, and will demonstrate the simple procedures necessary. It is best to practice the procedures you are shown on your cat while she is fit and healthy, and you are under no real pressure. An emergency situation is not the time to try out new procedures, as you will be under pressure and the cat may be in severe pain and therefore less than co-operative.

WARNING:
ALWAYS SEEK VETERINARY TREATMENT FOR A SICK OR AILING CAT.

Quick reference

Emergency techniques

The basics of first aid are as simple as ABC:

Airways **B**reathing **C**irculation

In other words, in emergency situations, the priority is to clear the cat's airway, to enable her to breathe, and to ensure that the blood is circulating properly, that is, the heart is beating. Then you can deal with any other symptoms.

Artificial respiration

If you find your cat unconscious in a collapsed state, the first requirement is to check that she is breathing. If there is little or no breathing, the cat's tongue will appear blue/black. If she is not breathing, check for foreign objects lodged in her mouth or throat, blocking her airways, and remove any blockages. Next, gently lift the cat's chin up to extend her neck, which will open up the cat's airway. If she is still not breathing, hold her mouth shut, and cover her nose with your mouth. Gently breathe up the cat's nose, giving approximately 30 breaths every minute. Keep this up until the cat begins breathing on her own, help arrives, or you believe the cat to be beyond help.

Chest compression

Next, check for a heartbeat. To do this, put your ear on the cat's chest, on the cat's left hand side, just behind her elbow. If the heart is beating, you should hear it. You can also check by putting your fingers in the same position. Another method of checking whether the heart is beating is to test for a pulse by placing two fingers on the inside of the cat's thigh, in the groin area.

If no heartbeat is present, you will need to begin chest compressions. To do this, place one hand on either side of the cat's chest, just behind her elbows, and squeeze the chest in a smooth action, giving two compressions

every second. Always use the flat of the hands and never the fingers. Also, be careful not to use too much force, as it is all too easy to break the cat's ribs.

Never attempt chest compressions if you suspect that the cat may have a chest injury.

Whichever method you use, give two breaths to the cat (artificial respiration) for about every four compressions. You must keep this up until the cat's heart begins to beat, or you cannot physically do any more, or a vet takes over from you. Keep checking for a heartbeat or a pulse throughout your attempts at heart massage.

Severe bleeding

Once you are certain that the cat is breathing and her heart is beating, any severe bleeding, or haemorrhage, must be controlled. Applying pressure, either directly or indirectly, or if the injury is on a limb, raising the limb, will help stem any blood flow. Use gauze, cotton wool or a clean handkerchief or piece of clothing to cover the wound and stem the flow. Direct pressure is simply pressure applied directly to the site of the bleeding, and can be done by squeezing the area in your hand, or holding a piece of cloth firmly to the affected area.

Never apply direct pressure to any wound with an object still impaled in it, or with a piece of bone protruding from it. In such circumstances, you will have to apply indirect pressure, either by applying pressure to the blood vessels above the wound (nearer to the heart) or by making a ring bandage and placing this around the object or bone, holding the ring bandage in place and applying pressure using another bandage or similar. A ring bandage is made by winding a piece of clean cloth (such as a triangular bandage) into a circle; the circle should be slightly larger than the area over which it is to be placed.

Most people are not used to seeing blood, and so tend to overestimate the amount

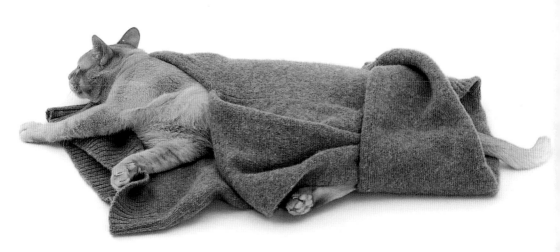

An unconscious cat should be covered with a towel or blanket to keep her warm while awaiting veterinary attention.

being lost. It is easy to panic at the sight of blood, but it is important to remain cool, calm and collected.

Never apply a tourniquet, since they can cut off the blood flow completely, causing severe – often life-threatening – danger to the patient.

The way in which the blood flows out of the wound will give you an idea of the type of blood vessel that is involved. Arteries carry blood from the heart to the organs and tissues. With one exception (the pulmonary artery, which passes blood from the heart to the lungs), all arteries carry oxygenated blood, which is extremely bright red, whereas the veins, again with one exception (the pulmonary vein, which passes blood from the lungs to the heart) carry de-oxygenated blood. Once the de-oxygenated blood is exposed to the atmosphere, the haemoglobin (which carries the oxygen in the blood) will become enriched with oxygen, thus turning the blood bright red. However, there can be no mistaking the way in which the different blood vessels actually bleed. The arteries carry blood under quite high pressure, as this blood comes directly from the heart. Any blood coming from an artery will therefore spurt out, whereas blood from the veins, under far less pressure, will flow smoothly. The blood vessels between the arteries and the veins, and which pass though organs and the skin, are called capillaries; capillary blood oozes slowly. Arterial blood will flow much faster than the other types, so will need to be attended to earlier. The type of bleeding will also be a good indication of the type and severity of the wound.

If any bleeding does not stop within five to ten minutes, veterinary treatment may be necessary. Any cat bleeding profusely must be taken to a vet immediately.

Serious injuries

THE ROLE OF THE FIRST AIDER
The priorities of the first aider are to:

● **Sustain life**
● **Prevent the victim's condition worsening**
● **Promote the victim's recovery**

Always remember to ensure your own safety at all times.

Immediate action in an emergency

In the event of an accident occurring, the first aider should do the following:

1 Assess the situation
Approach the injured cat carefully, looking for signs of injury and also any signs of danger to yourself or the cat. If the injured cat is in the middle of a road, consider moving her to a position safe for both the cat and yourself. Take care not to aggravate any injuries when moving a cat. Pick her up carefully, not putting any undue pressure on, or pulling, any area which may be injured. It is probably a good idea to use a garment or towel to restrain the cat safely (see p.109) as she will be frightened and in pain, making her more likely to bite. Speak to the cat throughout in a soft, calm voice, using her name if you know it.

Try to figure out what happened and what injuries the cat has sustained. Ask any witnesses to tell you what happened. This information will help you to decide how to deal with the situation.

2 Diagnose the cat's condition
If the cat seems to be unconscious, pinch her ear. If there is no response, the cat really is unconscious, and not just stunned. Look at her chest to see if she is breathing; if she is not, you must perform artificial respiration

(see p.104). You must then check that she has a heartbeat and if not, carry out chest compressions (see p.104). If she is breathing, consider whether she will require veterinary treatment, and if so, arrange for the vet to be contacted. You can always take the vet's advice on the situation, but do not allow this action to delay any life-saving action that may be needed on the spot.

3 Examine the cat
Check for any obvious injury, and make a note of its relative seriousness.

Check for bleeding, and treat accordingly (immediately and adequately (see p.104).

Check for any fractures, and treat accordingly (immediately and adequately (see p.113).

Check for any burns, and treat accordingly (immediately and adequately (see p.112).

Check the back of the cat's neck for 'lumps' and swellings. Any such lumps may indicate a broken bone, or swelling caused by injury. These symptoms will need to be passed on to the attending vet.

Finally, wait for the vet.

REMEMBER:
you must consider your own safety before attempting a rescue. Never risk your own life to try to save an injured cat, for example by running into a busy road. Always assess the situation before you attempt any rescue or begin any first aid work.

CHECKLIST OF ACTION POINTS

1 Always remember that your own safety is paramount.
2 Assess the situation.
3 Protect yourself and others from injury by the injured cat or traffic.
4 Examine the cat.
5 Diagnose injuries.
6 Treat injuries/treat for pain.
7 Keep the cat warm, calm and quiet.
8 If the injuries are serious, contact your ve*
9 Protect the cat from further injury.

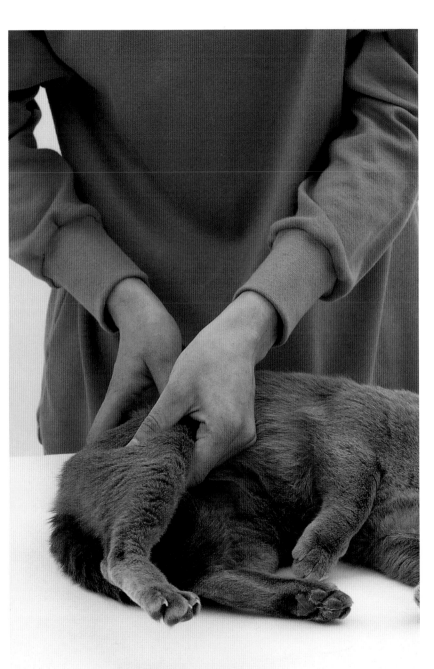

One of the best ways to take a cat's pulse is by placing two fingers on the inside of her rear thigh.

Specific injuries and conditions

Remember: an injured cat may object to being handled or even touched, and so you must be in a position to restrain her correctly (see p. 109).

BURNS

Minimize the damage from burns by cooling the burned area as quickly as possible with water (see p. 112).

OPEN WOUNDS

These must be covered with clean dressings to reduce the risk of infection.

UNCONSCIOUS CAT

Check for breathing and keep the airways open (see p. 104).

FRACTURES

Prevent further damage from broken bones by immobilizing the affected limb to avoid further movement and injury. (see p. 113).

BODY TEMPERATURE

It is extremely important that an injured cat is kept warm. If you have a 'space blanket', the cat should be wrapped in this. Failing a proper space blanket, use a sheet of 'bubble wrap', a coat or a jacket. If the cat is losing heat at a fast rate, or the surrounding temperature is extremely low, and it is necessary to try to warm the injured cat up, then you can cuddle her, sharing your own body heat with the cat. Never do this if there is any risk of the cat attacking you, unless you have restrained her (see below).

Moving and lifting an injured cat

You should not move any injured cat unless you have to, as any movement may aggravate her injuries. However, if you do need to move her, you should do this with great care. An injured cat may well object to being handled or even touched, so you must restrain her correctly. A cat has four feet, all equipped with razor-sharp claws, as well as a mouth full of very sharp teeth, all of which she may use to prevent you from holding her.

It is much easier to restrain, examine or treat a cat at about waist height, and so, if possible, the cat should be placed on a table or bench. First cover the surface of the table with a blanket or towel to help prevent the cat from slipping, which may cause her to panic. Once the cat is on the table, hold her firmly. The degree of restraint must be proportional to the procedure being carried out, the risk of the cat attacking the person treating her, and the cat's injuries.

A towel is useful to restrain a cat. Pick the cat up with one hand under her chest and the other under her rear end, spreading her weight, but ensuring that by doing so you will not be further aggravating any injury which she may have suffered. Once her feet are off

---

CLIPPING OF FUR AROUND WOUNDS

1 Using scissors with curved blades and rounded ends, and that have been dipped in water, carefully clip the fur around the wound. The clipped fur will stick to theblades of the scissors, preventing any from falling into the wound.
2 Dip the blades of the scissors in a bowl of water, and the clippings will come off in the water.

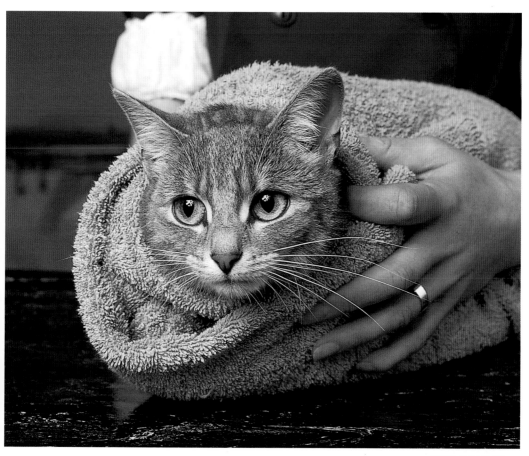

Before attempting to treat any injured cat, ensure that it is safely restrained, to prevent it from injuring you.

the ground, quickly cast the towel around her, ensuring that all four paws are within the folds of the towel. Throughout the time spent treating the cat's injuries, you should keep checking that she has not managed to extricate one or more paws.

Throughout any restraint, you must be firm but kind: talk quietly and calmly to the cat, offering her reassurance, and never frighten her by using too much force. To help ensure that your cat will always be fairly easy to restrain, practise restraint on her throughout her life, starting when she is a young kitten.

Major injuries and dangerous conditions

Bleeding

EXTERNAL
There are several different types of wound that a cat may suffer, and each requires slightly different treatment.

Minor wounds:
See p. 116 for the treatment of minor wounds.

Major wounds:
Clean (incised) cuts These are straight cuts, like one from a sharp knife blade. Bleeding, which may be profuse, helps clean the wound of debris, and this lessens the possibility of infection. Very often, incised cuts will bleed very little, if at all, even though the cut may be very deep, because the cut has not affected any major blood vessel. Any incised cut affecting the toes or a limb may cause damage to tendons, and so veterinary treatment should be sought. Many minor incised cuts will heal on their own, once they have been cleaned.

If possible, bleeding from an incised cut should be stemmed by direct pressure; if this is not possible, apply indirect pressure on an artery at the heart side of the wound. To find the artery, feel along the affected area, and you will be able to feel the vessel under the cat's skin. Elevating the injury will enable gravity to help reduce the blood flow. Apply a suitable dressing. Large and/or deep cuts will almost certainly require sutures (stitches) from a vet.
Lacerated cuts These are tears in the skin, such as those caused by barbed wire, for example, and bleed less profusely than incised cuts.
Puncture (stab) wounds Puncture wounds, which can be caused by nails, slivers of wood and other such objects, usually appear very small at the surface but, of course, could be very deep. *Never* remove any object from a wound, as this may aggravate the injury and/or allow large amounts of bleeding (while in place, such an object acts as a plug, and may be preventing massive blood loss). Apply pressure around the wound site, using a dressing to maintain the pressure, and seek veterinary advice immediately.
Gunshot wounds It is possible that your cat may be accidentally shot. If shot with a shotgun, the cat will be peppered with balls of shot (pellets), which will all require removal; bleeding should not be profuse. The vet will need to take an X-ray of the cat in order to locate all the pellets.

The other type of gunshot wound is from a bullet. Bullets make two wounds – an entry wound on the way in and an exit wound going out. Where 'sporting' (hollow point) ammunition is used, the exit wound will be several times larger than the entry wound. Where the bullet passes through any part(s) of the cat's anatomy, damage may be inflicted on any organ or tissue with which it comes into contact, and so all such wounds must be referred to a vet immediately. Air rifle pellets will have a similar effect, but are less likely to exit the cat's body.

In all cases of gunshot wounds, stem the flow of blood, keep the cat calm, checking for signs of trauma, and seek veterinary treatment immediately.

INTERNAL
Internal injuries are often manifested by swellings and bruising (contusions) in the cat's abdomen. Another sign of internal injuries is bleeding from the cat's mouth, eyes, ears, nose, anus or sex organs. A careful watch must be kept on the injured cat. Any cat showing any of these signs, or any signs of shock (see p.115) must be taken to a vet as soon as possible. Sometimes, the stools of a cat suffering from internal bleeding will be very dark reddish-brown.

Remember that the most common causes of bleeding from a queen's vulva are oestrus and cystitis (see p.36); oestrus, of course, does not require veterinary treatment.

Breathing problems

If your cat has stopped breathing, perform artificial respiration, see p.104.

Cats gasping for breath are obviously showing symptoms of some form of breathing difficulty; this may be heatstroke, fluid on the lungs or an obstruction of some kind in the airway. If the cat is suffering from heatstroke, she will appear very distressed, restless, and will pant a lot. If left untreated, her condition will rapidly deteriorate; she will drool and appear to be drunk, staggering around, completely unsteady on her feet. The treatment is to cool the cat down (see p.108).

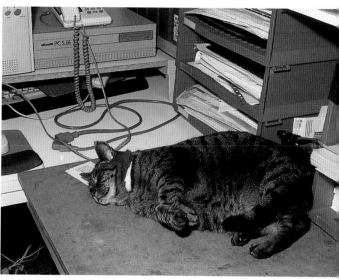

If you find your cat unconscious and not breathing, you must perform artificial respiration as soon as possible.

CHOKING:

Sometimes, a cat's breathing problems may be caused by something very simple, the most obvious cause being a blockage of the mouth or throat. If your cat suddenly appears to be choking, you must act immediately. To try to get her to a veterinary practice will waste time, and may result in her death. Take a secure hold on her and open her mouth to look inside and see if she has anything stuck in there. It is important that you have a good look in the cat's mouth before you start putting your fingers inside, as you may make matters worse by pushing a foreign object further down the throat. Very often, you will require assistance to remove an object blocking the mouth, so that one of you can hold open the cat's mouth to reduce the risk of the other being bitten. *Never* attempt to remove an object wedged in the cat's throat.

If you cannot remove the foreign object, you will need to take further, more drastic action. Holding the cat's hind legs, lift them over your knees, holding them between your knees. Placing one hand on either side of the chest, squeeze using jerky movements, making the cat 'cough'. Take care that you apply pressure proportional to the size of the cat: little pressure on a small kitten, more for a large adult cat. Squeeze about 5–6 times and the cat should cough out the lodged object.

Once the foreign object has been removed, you must let your cat rest, and take her to the vet for a check-up. If the foreign object is in the cat's throat or you cannot remove it from the mouth easily, you must obtain veterinary assistance urgently.

DROWNING:

On the whole, cats tend to avoid water, but they sometimes accidentally fall into ponds, streams and even rivers.

If your cat gets into difficulties while in water, ensure your own safety before making any rescue attempts.

Once she has been pulled from the water, she should be held upside down (if possible) to allow the water to drain from her lungs. Your cat will need veterinary treatment, and so someone should contact the vet as soon as possible. If you are on your own at the time of the emergency, shout to attract attention, and then ask anyone answering your calls to contact your vet and explain the situation.

Check that your cat is breathing. If she is not, you must begin artificial respiration, then check for a heartbeat and, if necessary, carry out chest compressions (see p.104). If luck is on your side, your cat should begin coughing and spluttering. Keep her quiet and calm. Rub her to dry off some of the water, and wrap her in a blanket or coat to keep her warm on her way to the vet.

Burns

There are two types of burn, one caused by heat and the other caused by chemicals.

HEAT BURNS:

The first treatment for any burn caused by heat, including scalds, is to reduce the heat, that is, cool the burn. This is best achieved by pouring cold water on the affected area. If you can stand the cat in a bath, run cold water on the affected area for at least ten minutes. The cooling will reduce the pain and the severity of the burn. Do not apply too much cold water at once, because too sudden a drop in the cat's temperature may cause more serious problems, and so her temperature should be reduced gradually.

While you are cooling the burned area, get someone to arrange for you to see the vet as soon as possible. Once you have cooled the affected area for at least ten minutes, cover the wound with a clean damp cloth, and wrap the injured cat in a space blanket or equivalent to keep her warm. If possible, get someone else to drive you to the vet, while you stay in the rear seat with the cat, to keep her calm and prevent her aggravating her injury.

CHEMICAL BURNS:

In the case of chemical burns, there is a danger of the cat ingesting the chemical if she licks the affected area, burning the inside of her mouth and throat etc. Wear rubber gloves to ensure that the chemical does not injure you. Thoroughly wash the affected area with running water, either by placing the cat in the bath and running water over the burn, or using a hose pipe in the garden.

While you are washing the affected area, get someone to arrange for you to see the vet as soon as possible. Once you have washed the affected area for at least ten minutes, cover the wound with a clean damp cloth, and wrap the injured cat in a space blanket or equivalent to keep her warm. If possible, get someone else to drive you to the vet, while you stay in the rear seat with the cat, to keep her calm and prevent her from licking the affected area or aggravating her injury.

Electrocution (electric shock)

A big danger in treating cats that have been electrocuted is the threat to the first aider. It is easy to rush in without considering any danger you might be in.

Whenever you suspect that a cat has been electrocuted, ensure that the power is switched off *before* you approach the injured cat. If it is not possible to switch off the power, do not approach the cat.

Once the power has been switched off and you are no longer in any danger, check that the cat is breathing. If she is not, begin artificial respiration, as detailed on p.104.

Electrocution will almost inevitably cause burns, which will need treating once the cat is breathing again (see p.112).

Fits and convulsions

Fits, convulsions and seizures are all the same, and are not a disease, but are symptoms of an underlying problem. There are many possible causes for convulsions, and two of the most common in cats are heatstroke (see p.113) and ingestion of slug pellets (see p.20). If a cat suffers regular, repeated fits, this may indicate that she is suffering from epilepsy (see p.98).

Do not attempt to hold down a fitting cat, but take care to limit how far the cat can move. If your cat is suffering from convulsions, you should seek urgent medical attention for her as seizures are extremely serious, and potentially life-threatening.

Fractures

Fractures (see p.42) are caused by either direct or indirect pressure on the bones, which may crack or actually break. Where the bone is broken and pierces the skin, this is known as an open or compound fracture; others are called closed fractures. Signs of such injury are obvious – painful movement of the limb, tenderness, swelling, loss of control of the limb, deformity of the limb, unnatural movement of the limb, and crepitus (the sensation or, in very bad cases, the sound of the two ends of the bones grinding on each other).

Keep the cat quiet, and steady and support the injured limb. Attempting to splint a fracture will cause the cat much pain, so it is best to leave this to the vet. Raising the limb will help reduce discomfort and swelling (by reducing the blood flow). A vet should treat any fracture as soon after the injury has taken place as possible.

Heatstroke

Cats cannot tolerate high temperatures and may die from heatstroke. Prevention is better than cure. Inside a car, the temperature can quickly rise to a dangerous level, even in the cooler sunshine of autumn and spring. If you leave your cat in a car for any period of time, particularly when the surrounding

temperature is high and/or there is a lot of sunshine, she may be dead on your return. No animal should be left unattended in a vehicle, or transported in full sunlight, without adequate ventilation. You must always remember that the sun does not stay in the same position throughout the day, so even if your car is in the shade when you leave it, it may be in the full sun later on. In extreme summer temperatures, or in areas where it is known that temperatures will be high, even more care must be taken than normal.

The first sign of heatstroke or heat exhaustion is an agitated cat in obvious distress. Affected cats may stretch out and pant heavily. The affected cat will start to drool and stagger around as if drunk; if left untreated, the cat will eventually collapse, pass into a coma and die.

Immediately a cat shows symptoms of heatstroke, you must act fast; delay can be fatal. The cat's body is overheating, so your first task is to lower her body temperature. With mildly affected cats, simply moving them to a cool area, and ensuring a steady passage

A cat with a fractured limb will not be easy to handle, and may well bite any person approaching her.

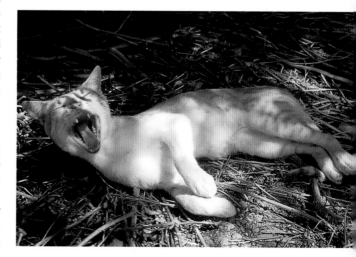

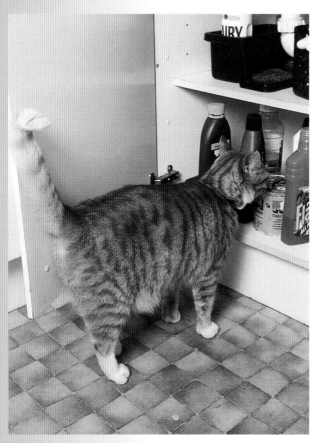

It is all too easy for cats to come into contact with the poisonous substances which are to be found in any home.

In bad cases, a hose pipe (on a fine misting spray) in the garden is effective. In very bad cases, cover the affected cat with wet towels (making sure that the mouth and nose are clear), and keep dousing the towels with cold water to keep them wet. Seek veterinary advice for all cats that are badly affected by heatstroke.

In all cases of heatstroke, it is vital to keep the head cool, as the brain may be quite literally cooked and brain death can occur.

Narcolepsy

A cat suffering from narcolepsy will appear to be extremely sleepy, although she will not lose consciousness. The condition is often associated with a condition known as cataplexy, where the affected cat will collapse and refuse to move. Some rat poisons also have this effect on a cat. If your cat shows any of these signs, you should consult the vet as soon as possible.

Poisoning

In cases of poisoning, it is most important to discover which poison your cat has taken. In the United Kingdom, with COSHH (the Control of Substances Hazardous to Health) Regulations, manufacturers must provide details of all substances that may be ingested. Businesses must also keep all such details of the substances that they use on the premises.

While you carry out any emergency procedures necessary, get someone to contact the vet, giving details of the poison that your cat has ingested if you know what it is. This will allow the practice time to get the relevant information from the manufacturer.

Do not make your cat vomit unless the manufacturer gives specific guidelines to do so.

If you are instructed to make the cat vomit, place a couple of washing soda (sodium

of cool air over them, is usually effective. Light spraying with cold water from a plant mister is also beneficial. If the cat is only suffering a mild case of heatstroke, once she has started to recover, ensure that she is thoroughly dried and placed in a cool area to recover fully.

carbonate) crystals on the back of the cat's tongue. If you have no washing soda, use mustard or salt in a strong solution. It is pointless to induce vomiting in a cat that has ingested a poison more than four hours earlier, as the substance will have passed through the stomach.

TYPES OF POISONING

Corrosive acids Car battery acid and the descaler used in central heating systems and kettles etc. are examples of corrosive acids. The acid must be neutralized as soon as possible, and the best way to do this is to get the cat to drink a solution of bicarbonate of soda (baking soda). The solution should be made up of half a teaspoon (approximately 2.5 ml) of sodium bicarbonate, dissolved in 250 ml (8 fl oz) of water. The sodium bicarbonate will dissolve better if the water is warm. Take the cat to the vet as soon as possible.

Never induce vomiting with corrosive acids.

Corrosive alkalis Creosote (used to treat fences and wooden kennels etc.) is the most common type of corrosive alkali likely to be ingested by a dog. Others may include paint stripper and oven cleaning fluids.

Again, the substance needs to be neutralized, by giving an acid solution (vinegar or orange juice) by mouth. Dilute the vinegar with an equal amount of water, though the orange juice can be given as it is.

Never induce vomiting with corrosive alkalis.

Irritants Irritants with which your cat may come into contact, and thus eat and ingest, include poisonous plants such as laburnum and poinsettia, or chemicals such as arsenic or lead. An extremely common source of cats suffering from 'poisoning', and one where they will be salivating profusely, is when the cat tries to eat a toad (*Bufo bufo*). The toad's skin is covered with pustules containing toxins designed to protect the creature from predators, and these toxins will affect the cat. Consult a vet immediately.

Narcotics Narcotic substances induce insensibility or stupor. Turpentine, paraffin and human sleeping tablets come under this category. Induce vomiting immediately if you have actually witnessed your cat eating narcotics, but if you are not certain when she may have eaten the substance, *do not induce vomiting*. If the narcotic has been in the cat's system for some time, it may be affecting her swallowing reflex, and if so, she may inhale her own vomit, with serious consequences.

If at all possible, keep the affected cat awake until she can be treated by a vet.

Convulsants Convulsants cause fits, which are involuntary actions of voluntary muscles. Slug pellets are the most likely convulsant for a cat to have ingested, but she may have eaten laurel or anti-freeze (ethylene glycol). If you know that your cat has definitely taken these substances, induce vomiting immediately, and seek veterinary guidance and advice urgently.

Shock

Shock, which is an acute fall in blood pressure, is often evident after the cat has been involved in an accident or has been injured; certain diseases can also cause this condition. The symptoms of shock include cool skin, pale lips and gums (due to the lack of circulation); faint, rapid pulse; staring but unseeing eyes.

The cat must be kept warm and the blood circulation returned to normal as soon as possible. Massaging the cat will help to improve her circulation, and wrapping her in a towel or blanket will help keep her warm. Be careful that by doing this you do not cause more damage by aggravating any injuries such as fractures or cuts. The affected cat should be kept quiet and warm, and veterinary treatment sought as soon as possible.

Minor Injuries

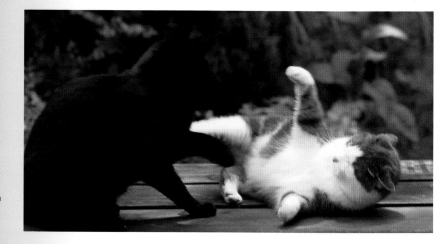

Many cats suffer from being attacked and bitten by other cats, in the course of their everyday activities.

Bites and stings

There are four types of bite and sting: cat, insect, rat and snake.

CAT BITES

Cats are more likely to suffer from bites from other cats than from any other animal, especially as most cats are allowed to wander. Such cats are regularly involved in fights with other cats.

It is unlikely that you will be present when your cat is fighting, but if you are, you will be tempted to stop the fight. Before attempting to break up a fight between two or more cats, ensure your own safety. A long-handled sweeping brush or broom will help drive off the other cats, and also keep them far enough away from you to prevent you being bitten. If to hand, a bucket of cold water, or water sprayed from a hose pipe, will be extremely effective, stopping the cats from fighting, and also giving you the opportunity to get them under control.

If a bite has caused only minor injuries, the area of the bite should be clipped of fur, ensuring that the clippings do not become entangled in the wound itself. Wetting the scissors is recommended, as the hairs stick to the blades rather than falling onto the wound; dipping the scissors into a jug of water after each snip will remove all hairs from the metal. The wound should then be thoroughly washed with a saline solution followed by an antiseptic liquid. Finally, give the area a good dusting with an antiseptic wound powder. If action is not taken, the wound may fester and result in abscesses. Cat bites almost always end up infected if not treated adequately.

INSECT BITES (including stings)

Clip a little fur away from the area, so that you can actually see the problem, then wash with saline solution. Bees leave their sting in the victim, wasps do not. If there is a sting present, it should be carefully removed with the tweezers and then the area wiped with cotton wool (or a cotton bud) soaked in alcohol, such as surgical spirit. For wasp stings, a little vinegar will prove beneficial while for bee stings, use a little bicarbonate of soda (the stings are alkaline, and the vinegar or bicarbonate of soda neutralizes the effect of the sting). Dry the area thoroughly, and apply a wet compress to help reduce the irritation and swelling.

If the cat has been bitten or stung in the throat, seek veterinary attention as soon as possible; such stings can cause swelling that may block the airways and kill the cat.

RAT BITES

Rat bites are some of the most dangerous bites that a cat may suffer. Rats can carry many very harmful diseases and their teeth are dirty so there is a good chance the wounds will become infected.

The area of the wound should be clipped of fur, then thoroughly cleaned with a saline solution and then an antiseptic liquid; dry and apply liberal amounts of antiseptic (antibiotic) dusting powder. All cats bitten by rats should be taken to the vet as soon as possible after the injury, where the vet may administer an injection of antibiotics. An antibiotic dusting powder may be prescribed for the wound.

SNAKE BITES

There are many venomous snakes, although only one species, the adder (*Vipera berus*) lives in the United Kingdom. It is unusual for cats to be bitten by these reptiles but it does sometimes happen.

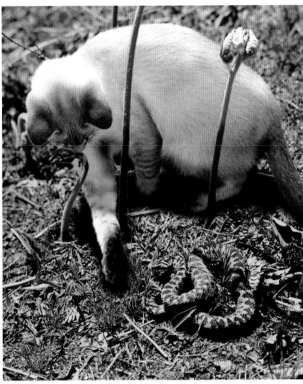

Above: **In areas where venomous snakes may be encountered, it is not unusual for cats to attack them and be bitten in the process.**

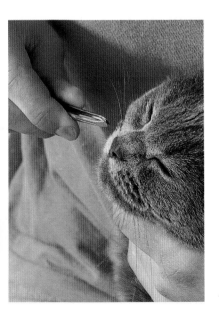

Left: **Bee stings should be carefully removed from the injured cat, and the area then cleaned.**

During the spring or early summer, snakes are rather lethargic, especially the gravid (pregnant) females; this is due to the cool temperatures, since snakes are exothermic and require external heat to warm their bodies to their preferred body temperature. At such time, while they are warming themselves, they will keep still for as long as possible, even when approached. If your cat sees a snake and decides to attack it, or she stands on it, the snake will bite.

It is extremely important that you keep the injured cat as calm as possible and prevent her from running around, or even making any movements, as this will speed up the circulation of the venom around the cat's body. You must also remain calm, as your actions will influence the cat. Seek immediate veterinary attention.

Minor bleeding

The big danger with any cuts is that the injury will have pushed dirt and debris into the wound, and unless there is a great deal of bleeding the dirt will not be washed out. Clean the wound with saline solution (two teaspoonfuls (approximately 10 ml) of salt to 1 litre (1¾ pints)of warm water); dry it, apply an antiseptic ointment or cream, and apply a dressing if necessary.

Broken teeth

Cats, like humans, can damage their teeth, making eating extremely painful (see p.22). Broken teeth are often accompanied by bleeding from the cat's mouth. Broken teeth must be treated by the vet.

Severe diarrhoea

Every reader will recognize the signs of diarrhoea, and also realize that this may simply be a symptom of over-eating. However, it may also be a symptom of more serious problems (see p.30).

In all cases of severe diarrhoea, where over-eating is definitely not the cause, you should prevent your cat eating anything and contact the vet. You should also contact the vet if there is blood in the feces. It is essential that your cat is provided with ample drinking water or, even better, give her re-hydrating fluid. Keep your cat where you can see her, covering the floor with newspapers or similar to keep your home clean, and note the times of her motions, and also the consistency, colour and quantity of the diarrhoea. By doing this, you will help the vet to find the cause of the sudden diarrhoea, and thereby treat the problem effectively.

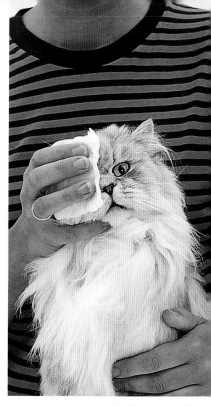

A cold compress will help soothe a swollen eye. Do not let the cat rub the affected eye, it may exacerbate the injured eye.

Eye injury

Any injury to the eye can cause serious damage to the cat's sight, so any eye injuries must be seen by the vet (see pp.48–55).

If your cat has an injured eye she will be holding it half closed, and the eye itself will be swollen and/or bleeding. The cat will probably be trying to rub her affected eye, and this should not be allowed, as it may aggravate the injury.

See p.111 for how to deal with foreign objects in the eye.

If the eye is swollen, the gentle application of a cold compress (a cold, wet cloth) may be beneficial. However, do *not* apply any bandage or compress if you suspect that there may be a foreign body in the eye, as this may cause further damage.

Fainting

This is a loss of consciousness caused by a sudden lack of blood supply to the brain. It can also be caused by low blood sugar levels. Treat her as unconscious (see p.108), and take her to the vet as soon as possible.

Foreign bodies

Most cats are inquisitive, and tend to lead lifestyles that may occasionally lead them to pick up items that they really should not. Consequently, foreign bodies may become lodged in various parts of their anatomy.

IN THE ANUS

A cat that has swallowed a foreign object that her body cannot digest may pass the object out of her anus. Often, this occurs without any problem, and without the owner even knowing about it. Occasionally, however, the object may be seen hanging half out of the anus; the owner must attempt to remove the object without hurting the cat. As most cats do not take well to interference in this area, it is wise to take the precaution of adequately restraining the cat before you start to try to remove the foreign object.

Once the cat is suitably restrained, carefully examine the foreign object and, unless it appears sharp, gently pull it. If there is any resistance to your pulls, stop immediately, and take the cat to the vet for help.

IN THE EYE

The cat will probably be trying to rub her affected eye, and this should not be allowed, as it may aggravate the injury, so you must physically restrain her.

Holding the cat's head very steady, and using a magnifying lens, you can look in the eye for any foreign object (such as a grass seed or small piece of hay). Often, such objects get stuck behind the eyelid (either upper or lower). This procedure is often best left for the vet, as it is all too easy to damage the cat's eye.

If any foreign object is seen, do not try to remove it with fingers, tweezers or similar objects, as this may lead to serious and irreparable eye damage. Instead, use warm water, and gently and slowly pour it over the affected eye, while the eyelids are held open. This action may flush the object out.

IN THE NOSE

Unless you are certain the foreign object is very short, do not attempt to remove it from your cat's nose. Contact the vet immediately.

IN A WOUND

Never remove any foreign object from a wound. To do so may aggravate the wound, and cause further bleeding. Seek veterinary treatment.

Lameness

A cat that is unable to bear her weight on one or more of her legs, or is unable to walk, is described as lame. The condition is covered in detail on p.41.

If your cat suddenly becomes lame, contact the vet as soon as possible, and keep the cat still and resting until the vet can examine her.

Vomiting

Vomiting is a muscular reflex action, resulting in expulsion, under force, of the contents of the cat's stomach and/or small intestine (see p.28). It is quite normal for a cat to vomit small amounts occasionally, and only if the cats vomits two or three times within a short period should you consult the vet.

If your cat does vomit a few times within a short period, prevent her from eating or drinking anything, and contact the vet. Keep your cat where you can see her, covering the floor with newspapers or similar to keep your home clean, and note the times of vomiting, and also the consistency, colour and quantity of the vomit. By doing this, you will help the vet to find the cause of the sudden vomiting, and thereby treat the problem effectively.

The first aid kit

Some of the most common cat injuries – minor cuts and abrasions – occur when the cat is going about its daily routine, and it is important that they are treated as soon as possible. In order to do this, you should have a small first aid kit. You should, of course, also have the necessary skill and experience to treat these minor injuries, and you can get advice from your vet on various minor procedures. If there is any doubt as to the seriousness of the injuries, or the cat's general condition, consult the vet as soon as possible: they will be happy to advise you on the best course of action.

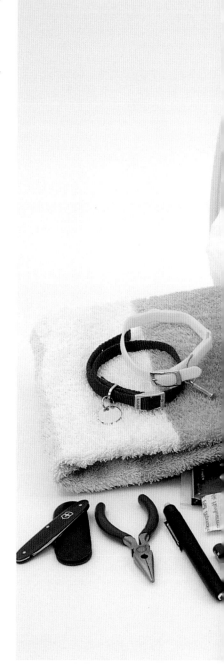

Contents of a cat first aid kit

A good first aid kit may even save your cat's life. It is, however, vital that you know exactly how to use all the items. A good book such as this one is also useful, and should be kept close to the first aid kit.

The following are all items that should be included in a first aid kit, which you should have near at hand at all times. Do not forget to replace any item you use straight away, before it is needed again. Many of the items listed in this kit can be used on either cat or human injuries.

1 ALCOHOL (surgical spirit)
For the removal of ticks etc. (see p.68).

2 ANTIHISTAMINE
For the treatment of insect stings (see p.116). It comes as cream or lotion, and can be purchased from the vet or a pharmacy.

3 ANTISEPTIC LOTION
For cleaning cuts, wounds and abrasions. Soap and water or brine (salt and water solution made with 2 teaspoonfuls (10 ml) salt to 1 litre (1¾ pints) of water) is as good as antiseptic lotion.

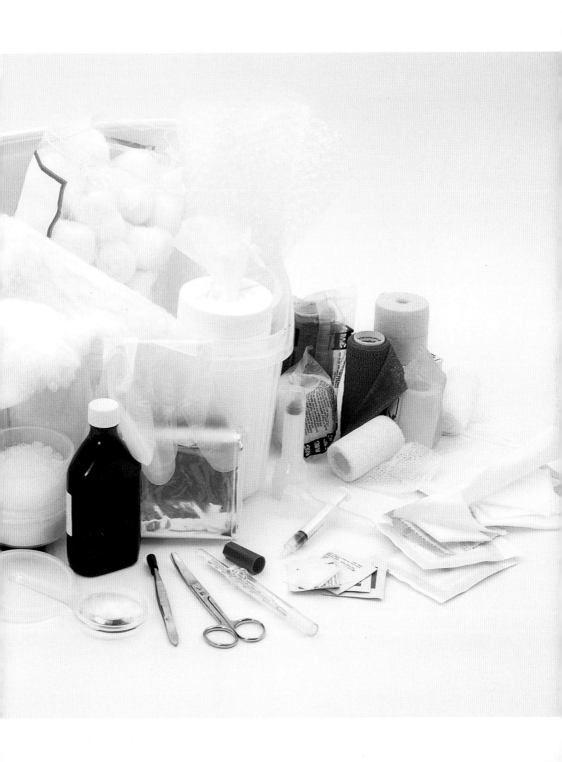

4 BANDAGES

For binding broken limbs and wounds. Keep a selection of small bandages. They will only be temporary, as the cat will chew them off.

5 COTTON BUDS

For cleaning wounds and applying ointments etc. With care, they can also be used to clean the ear flaps but *under no circumstances* should you poke these (or any other object) into the ear canal.

6 COTTON WOOL

For cleaning wounds, cuts and abrasions, and for stemming the flow of blood. Dampen all cotton wool before use with tap water, otherwise strands will stick to the wound, causing possible complications.

7 ELIZABETHAN COLLAR

Useful to (try to!) prevent a cat from interfering with dressings, sutures etc. It is simple to make one of these using an old plastic bucket by splitting it and cutting a hole in the centre, of a size to fit comfortably around the cat's neck. You could also use a piece of strong cardboard.

8 EYE WASH

For washing out debris from a cat's eyes. It is also advisable to obtain some local anaesthetic, sold at pharmacists for relieving the pain of eye injuries, until veterinary treatment can be obtained for the injured cat.

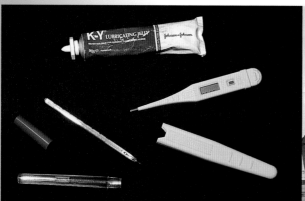

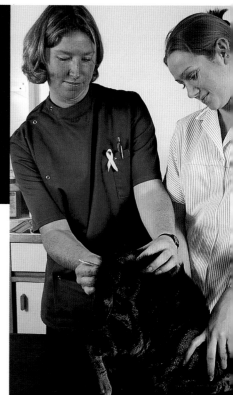

Above: **Types of clinical thermometer suitable for use on cats. The KY jelly is a lubricant.**

Right: **Many injuries will require the cat to be examined by the vet.**

9 KAOLIN PECTATE

For use in cases of diarrhoea. Available from any vet, a pharmacy or even from many supermarkets. Follow the dosage recommendations on the label. Veterinary advice will be given when it is dispensed.

10 KY JELLY

A lubricant that should be applied to a thermometer before it is inserted into the cat's rectum. It is available from a pharmacist or a vet. If KY jelly is not available, petroleum jelly or even liquid soap or washing-up liquid may be used.

11 NAIL CLIPPERS

For trimming the cat's nails. These should be top quality. Use the type that work on the guillotine principle, where one blade hits the other, rather than on the scissors principle, which can result in nails being pulled out.

12 RECTAL THERMOMETER

For taking the cat's temperature. Modern thermometers are electronic, making a 'beep' when they have been in position long enough to take the cat's temperature, and they have a digital read-out.

13 SCISSORS

For cutting the fur away around any wound. These should be curved and round-ended. They must *not* be used for trimming the cat's nails.

14 SPACE BLANKET

To help maintain the cat's body temperature. This is a large sheet of aluminium foil, available at camping and hiking shops. A suitable, though more bulky alternative, is a large sheet of 'bubble wrap'. The blanket must be large enough to cover the cat adequately.

15 STYPTIC PENCIL

To help stem the flow of capillary blood, for example from very minor cuts or bleeding claws. Available from pharmacists (sold to stem blood flow in humans). Be warned that this will sting the cat, who is likely to react accordingly!

16 SURGICAL GAUZE

For padding wounds and stemming the flow of blood.

17 TABLE SALT

For making into solution. Two teaspoons (approximately 10 ml) of salt mixed in 1 litre (1¾ pints) of warm water is a good solution with which to wash debris from wounds and counter infection. One teaspoon (approximately 5 ml) of salt mixed in 1 litre (1¾ pints) of warm water with one tablespoon of glucose makes an excellent re-hydrating fluid for cats. Glucose is a simple sugar, available in powder form from any pharmacy or health food store. The fluid should be given to the cat to drink instead of her normal water. If she will not drink, use a syringe, and put the solution directly into the cat's mouth, as you would if you were administering a liquid medicine.

18 TOWEL

No matter how tame you believe your cat to be, when she is in pain she may bite or scratch anyone who comes close, particularly when that person is handling the injured area. It is best always to err on the side of safety and to restrain any injured cat before beginning examination or treatment. A towel is useful to wrap around the cat, in order to restrain her safely, and prevent her from injuring anyone (see p.108).

19 TWEEZERS (forceps)

For the removal of foreign bodies. Ensure that these have rounded ends to minimize the chance of injuring the cat. Different lengths may be useful.

index

acknowledgements

The Feline Centre and the Feline Advisory Bureau 15 Top, 15 Bottom, 53, 79.
Sylvia Cordaiy/Anthony Reynolds 116.
David A. Crossley 11, 17, 18, 29, 45.
John Daniels 4 Top, 12, 14, 32, 34 Top Right, 47, 48, 60, 68, 94, 96, 117 left.
Frank Lane Picture Agency/David Hosking 9 Bottom Left, /Life Science Images 30 /Martin B Withers 42.
Octopus Publishing Group Ltd. 6–7, 67 Bottom Left, /Jane Burton 26 Bottom Left, 91, 118, 120–121, /Paul Bus 58, /Robert Estall 34 Bottom Left, /Rosie Hyde 4–5, 38, /Dick Polak 109, /Ron Sutherland 90.
Angela Hampton/Family Life Picture Library 24, 51, 61 Top, 69 right, 72, 74, 83, 93, 122 right.
Jacana/Jean Paul Thomas 87 right.
James McKay 122 left.
Veterinary Dermatology Service/Sue Paterson 67 Top Right.
RSPCA Photolibrary 9 Top Right, /Jane Burton 97 Top Right, /Angela Hampton 20, 21, 26 Top Right, 33, 35 right, 64, 66, 70, 75, 88, 98, 113, 114, /Stuart Harrop 56, /Mike Lane 111, /Ken McKay 10, /Stephen Oliver 39, /Alan Robinson 3, /Marie Sterner 76.
Science Photo Library/Eye of Science 25, /Moredun Animal Health LTD 97 left /Dr Linda Stannard, UCT 31.
Warren Photographic/Jane Burton 8, 13, 16, 23 Top, 23 Bottom, 35 left, 36, 37, 40, 41, 44, 46, 49, 50, 52, 54, 59 Top, 59 Bottom, 61 Bottom, 62, 63, 65, 71 Top, 71 Bottom, 73, 80, 81, 82, 84, 86, 87 left, 89, 101, 102–103, 105, 107, 117 right, /Kim Taylor 55, 69 left.